URINARY SEDIMENT: A TEXTBOOK ATLAS

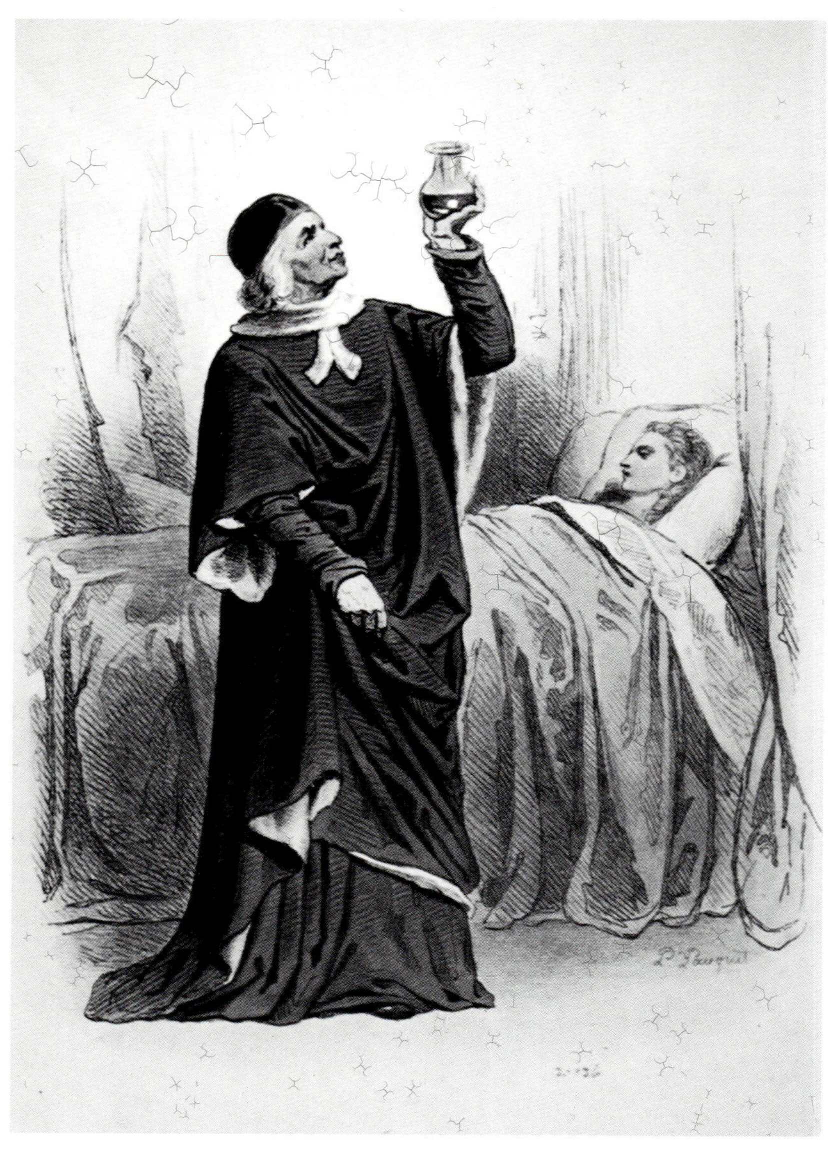

This is a 19th century French lithograph copied from an illustration in a 13th century illuminated medical manuscript. Physicians of the Middle Ages examined urine in special flasks for prognostication, and it was not until modern times when the sediment was examined chemically and microscopically that the art became a science.

URINARY SEDIMENT: A TEXTBOOK ATLAS

Meryl H. Haber, MD

Professor, Department of Pathology, Rush Medical College, Chicago; Former Professor and Chairman, Department of Laboratory Medicine and Pathology, and Medical Director, Medical Technology Program, University of Nevada School of Medicine, Reno

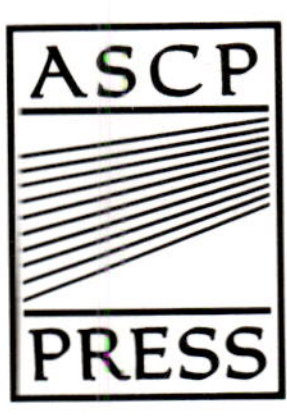

Educational Products Division
American Society of Clinical Pathologists
Chicago

Library of Congress Cataloging in Publication Data

Haber, Meryl H., 1934–
Urinary sediment: a textbook atlas

Bibliography: p.
Includes index.
1. Urine—Examination—Atlases. I. Title. [DNLM:
1. Urine—Analysis—Atlases. QY 17 H114u]
RB53.H25 616.07'566 81–4413
ISBN 0–89189–103–X AACR2

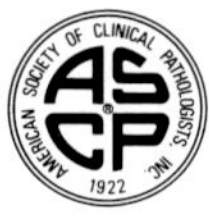

Printed in Hong Kong by Everbest Printing Co., Ltd.

Reprinted in 1983, 1989, 1991, 1994.

CONTRIBUTORS

Donald C. Cannon, MD, PhD

Pathologist, Professional Medical Laboratories, Wichita Falls, Texas

Luther E. Lindner, MD, PhD

Assistant Professor of Pathology, Texas A and M University, College Station, Texas

Dyan Monte-Verde, MT (ASCP), MS

Clinical Information System Representative and Educator, Ames Company, Division of Miles Laboratories, Rochester, New York

Anne Thompson, MT (ASCP), SH

Administrative Director of Laboratory, North Trident Regional Hospital, Charleston, South Carolina

To my fellow laboratory
workers from whom I have received
much more than I have given

In the investigation of diseases at the bedside, the physician is called upon to avail himself not only of every general symptom presented by the patient, but of every indication afforded by the secretions and excretions; and among those guides to a correct diagnosis, an examination of the urine is of essential importance.

Golding Bird, AM, MD, *Urinary Deposits, Their Diagnosis, Pathology, and Therapeutical Indications*, 1844

CONTENTS

ILLUSTRATIONS

KEY: BF = bright-field microscopy, PH = phase-contrast microscopy, ICM = interference-contrast microscopy, and Pol = polarized microscopy.

PREFACE

In undertaking the writing and editing of this textbook atlas, it was my intention to present a clinically useful book about urinary sediment that would ultimately serve as both a teaching tool and reference source. Realizing the difficulties of the task at hand, especially in regard to limitations imposed by production costs, it was necessary to be highly selective in choosing the topics and illustrations. However, I felt that for this atlas to be most helpful and meaningful, nothing could supplant color photomicrographs. For this reason, color is used extensively to represent sediment elements as they are actually seen by the microscopist, and with the hope that the color photomicrographs will be more meaningful in the clinical interpretation of urinary sediments than the ordinary black-and-white format.

To add to the didactic value of the book, I included a chapter on quality assurance and also one on scanning electron microscopy (SEM) of the sediment. To appreciate fully the significance of the urinary sediment in clinical diagnosis, one must be assured that data obtained from this examination are both precise and accurate. In my estimation, there is no way to obtain meaningful information without establishing quality assurance standards in every laboratory in which urinalyses are performed. Therefore, Chapter 10 was inserted not as an absolute but as a guideline that can be adapted to serve the needs of various laboratories. I would like to emphasize that the urinalysis section of a laboratory should be treated like any other specialized area within the same laboratory; more specifically, all specimens submitted for examination should be handled similarly and with appropriate controls so that the results are both accurate and meaningful. The chapter on scanning electron microscopy was selected to promote interest in the subject matter. Certainly, it is not expected that SEM examination of urinary sediments should become a routine procedure in pathology laboratories. However, as one can see by the photographs in this chapter, the ability to view the sediment at higher magnifications using the SEM technique enhances interest in the subject matter and also enables the observer to define and appreciate the composition of the sediment elements.

It is hoped that this atlas will be used as a primary reference source as well as a working text for physicians, technologists, and students engaged in urine sediment examination or its study. It is also meant to show that urinalysis is a dynamic and important field of medicine and should not be overlooked or subjected to a "backroom" approach. Physicians throughout the ages such as Hippocrates, Paracelsus, and Richard Bright have advocated the use of urinalysis and its importance in clinical diagnosis. I would also like to make the same recommendation. As a step in that direction, this atlas was designed to help the reader examine and interpret urine sediment with a greater degree of confidence and accuracy than heretofore possible.

MERYL H. HABER, MD

ACKNOWLEDGMENTS

During the many years of studying urinary sediment, I have received invaluable assistance and advice from numerous professional colleagues. To them a great debt is owed. In addition, I am grateful to several other experts in the field for their assistance in writing chapters and compiling photomicrographs that are interspersed throughout the text.

I would like to thank the following persons for contributing their photomicrographs to this atlas:

Donald C. Cannon, MD, PhD—Figures 2–17, 2–21, 3–3, 5–7, 5–26, 5–27, 5–30, 6–36, 6–37, 8–3 through 8–7, 9–1 through 9–7, 9–10, and 9–12.

Luther E. Lindner, MD, PhD—Figures 6–52, 6–53, 6–55, and 7–1 through 7–10.

Dyan Monte-Verde, MT (ASCP), MS—Figures 2–31, 5–23, 5–25, 5–29, 5–31, 5–32, and 6–56.

Anne Thompson, MT (ASCP), SH—Figures 2–8, 2–27, 5–1, 5–4, 5–5, 5–8, 5–9, 5–10, 5–13, 5–14, 5–17 through 5–20, 5–22, and 5–24.

Finally, I wish to thank my secretary, Mary Barnewitz, for her cooperation and assistance in the organization and typing of the manuscript.

MHH

1. INTRODUCTION

NORMAL URINARY SEDIMENT

The urinary sediment of human beings may contain a wide variety of substances or elements.[1, 21, 28] These elements have various origins and may be metabolic products of the kidney, such as crystals; cells derived from the bloodstream or urinary tract; cells from other organs of the body, such as spermatozoa from the testes; and various proteinaceous substances that have their origin in the kidney, such as casts. In addition, other elements are frequently found in the urine of patients without apparent renal disease that are not human in origin and that appear as contaminants. The most common of these are bacteria and yeasts. A wide variety of artifacts and exogenous materials, such as talc, man-made fibers, and pollen grains, must be recognized for what they are, as an inexperienced observer might easily misdiagnose these substances as abnormal sediment elements.

The most important consideration in the microscopic examination of the urine sediment is to distinguish the contents of the normal sediment from the abnormal. At best, normality of the urine is a feature of health and, to the examining physician, an indicator that the urinary tract is functioning properly and not producing elements that may be indicators of disease. The most significant distinguishing feature of normality is, in most cases, simply the presence of limited numbers of certain elements and the absence of others.[3] For example, white and red blood cells derived from the bloodstream are found in small numbers in the sediment of healthy persons. However, when blood cells are found in larger numbers in the sediment, this is considered an abnormal condition.

To determine whether or not a specific increase of any one or a number of sediment elements is present, and whether or not this increase is expected or is a true or real increase indicating a pathologic disease of the urinary tract, the observer must be certain that the results obtained when performing the sediment examination are precise, accurate, and reproducible.[21] In Chapter 10 quality assurance is discussed in relation to examination of the urinary sediment. However, at this point it cannot be stressed too strongly that for meaningful results to be obtained—results that ensure a high level of quality in care, in both diagnosis and therapy—the urinoscopist must initiate procedures in the laboratory that promote accurate recognition and diagnosis of disease states.

Not only is it important to be able to distinguish the abnormal sediment from the normal on the basis of numbers of elements present alone; one must also be able to recognize any variations that might occur in the "normal" sediment. The most typical example of such variation is that which occurs under stressful conditions.[49] Studies have shown that when a normal person is under stress, the urine sediment will abruptly be altered, with the appearance of hyaline and granular casts in abnormal numbers.[23] It behooves the observer to be aware of such alterations in the normal state and to communicate these findings to the attending physician in an appropriate context.

An additional facet that must be considered in the evaluation of the urinary sediment is that of distinguishing any "normal" elements present from possible artifacts that may easily be confused with pathologic elements. I refer to such things as scratches on the underside of coverslips, which may be confused with urine casts; the clumping or accumulation of crystalline matter, which may also be mistaken for casts; air bubbles, which are commonly misdiagnosed as urinary lipids; and numerous other particulate matter, such as vegetable cells, plant fibers, talcum granules, and skin oil droplets, which may be confused with various pathologic sediment elements.

The tools that the urinoscopist uses in a day-to-day working existence are relatively simple and consist predominantly of an ordinary light microscope equipped with an optical system, which must provide optimal conditions of light to enhance contrast and capitalize on small differences of density present in the elements viewed. Various forms of optical enhancement have been advocated over the past decade. Among these are the addition to the usual bright-field optical system of phase-contrast[11, 56] and interference-contrast microscopy equipment.[4, 18, 19] Both phase-contrast and interference-contrast microscopy capitalize on the differences in physical properties of sediment elements showing changes in refractive index. Both types of microscopy are now widely used in urinalysis laboratories. Throughout this text results using both of these techniques will be illustrated, since they enhance sediment element recognition and provide a specific visual means of increasing diagnostic capability. In addition, supravital staining of the urinary sediment also enhances recognition of elements.

ABNORMAL URINARY SEDIMENT

The urinoscopist must be able to distinguish the contents of the abnormal urinary sediment.[12, 21] To do this adequately, the limits of the normal must be known. However, a quantitative measurement of the number and type of sediment elements present in the normal urine is not sufficient. The urinoscopist must, in addition, be able to recognize specifically various abnormal sediment elements that are not present in normal urine. These elements are widely diverse in nature. Among the most important and also the most commonly observed are various forms of casts; certain crystals indicating abnormalities in bodily metabolism; and other components, such as parasites, that involve the urinary tract of man.

This atlas is by no means intended to be encyclopedic in either its textual content or its illustrations, which depict the various types of sediment elements. However, a wide variety of both normal and abnormal urinary contents are illustrated, and the reader is supplied with sufficient examples of each so that ultimately specific distinctions can be made among normal, abnormal, and artifactual elements.

A word of caution now needs to be interjected in regard to the diagnosis of urine sediment elements. This text will demonstrate the importance of the microscopic examination of the urine sediment in patient diagnosis and quality care. It therefore goes without saying that a competent and well trained microscopist must be given responsibility for the urinalysis section of a clinical laboratory. Only in this way can accurate diagnosis be done. In addition, the equipment housed in that section of the laboratory should be kept clean and be of a relatively high degree of quality and sophistication. With the appropriate tools at hand, the urinoscopist will have no difficulty recognizing any elements present in the urinary sediment and communicating their importance to the attending physician. Each and every laboratory should be concerned with quality of care and work for the good of the patient. Also, as new methods, instruments, and techniques evolve that affect the urinalysis section of the laboratory, they should be applied promptly and expeditiously to ensure quality care.

2. CELLS OF THE URINARY SEDIMENT

EPITHELIAL CELLS

Three main varieties of epithelial cells, all derived from the epithelial lining of the kidney and lower urinary tract, are found in the urine. These cells may be distinguished from one another by the trained examiner.[30] In addition, those cells lining the renal nephrons may be selectively stained by histochemical techniques, when appropriate, to identify their exact site of origin in the renal tubule (ie, proximal or distal tubule). A brief discussion of the morphologic characteristics of each epithelial cell types follows, and cellular contents of normal urinary sediment are presented in Table 2–1.

TABLE 2–1.—Cellular Contents of Normal Urinary Sediment

CELL TYPE	SIZE, μ	SHAPE	OTHER CHARACTERISTICS
Epithelial cells			
Squamous	30–50	Flat	Nucleus 7–12 μ
Transitional	20–30	Spheric or tadpole	Syncytia
Renal	15–25	Polyhedral	Microvillous border
Other	13–25	Cuboidal to columnar	Corpora amylacea-associated, clumps
Blood			
Red cells (erythrocytes)	7.5	Biconcave	Crenated
White cells (leukocytes)	12–15	Spheric	PMNs, granules, motile
Spermatozoa	45–60	Tadpole	Motile, head 4–6 μ

Squamous Epithelial Cells

These are the largest of all cells found in the urinary sediment and the easiest to recognize morphologically (Figs 2–1 through 2–3). They measure between 30 and 50 μ in cross diameter; are flattened; and have a central, small, spheric, and condensed nucleus. The nuclear diameter is approximately that of a red blood cell (7.5 μ). The cytoplasm of squamous cells is normally smooth, but may be wrinkled, depending on the osmolarity of the urine and whether or not the cells have had an opportunity to dry or become altered because of standing.

When urine has been left at room temperature for long periods of time before microscopic evaluation, squamous epithelial cells in the urine undergo degenerative changes (Fig 2–4). The cytoplasm may appear granular, and the nucleus and cyto-

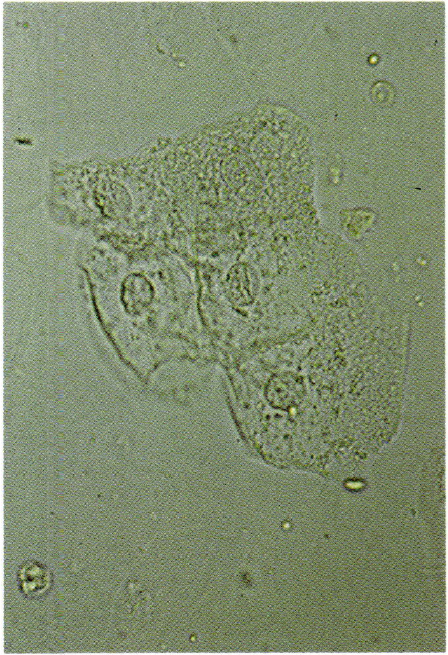

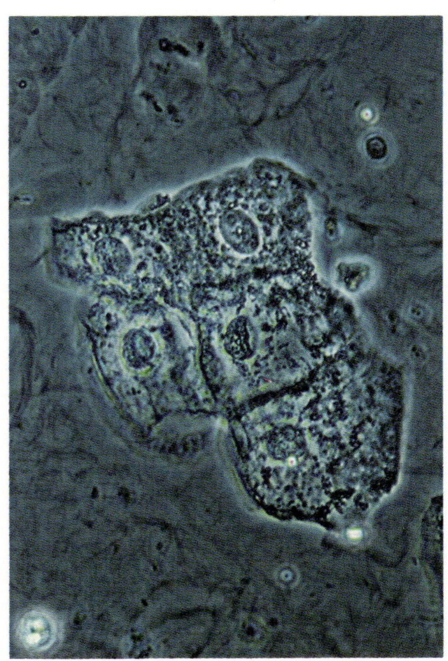

Fig 2–1 ***(left).*** Squamous epithelial cells, commonly seen in clumps, but also singly. They are large, flat, and often have finely wrinkled cytoplasm (BF ×200).

Fig 2–2 ***(right).*** Group of squamous epithelial cells with mucus strands in the background. Here, the difference between phase-contrast (PH) and bright-field (BF) microscopy is demonstrated (PH ×200).

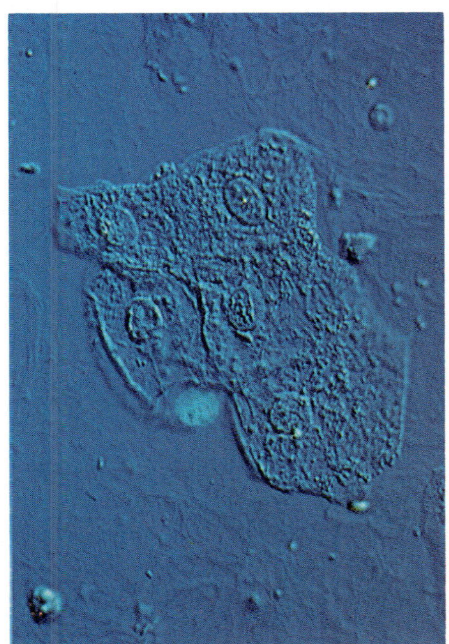

Fig 2–3. Group of squamous epithelial cells, characterized by fine granularity and wrinkling. Interference-contrast microscopy enhances surface characteristics by providing a relief or three-dimensional image (ICM ×200).

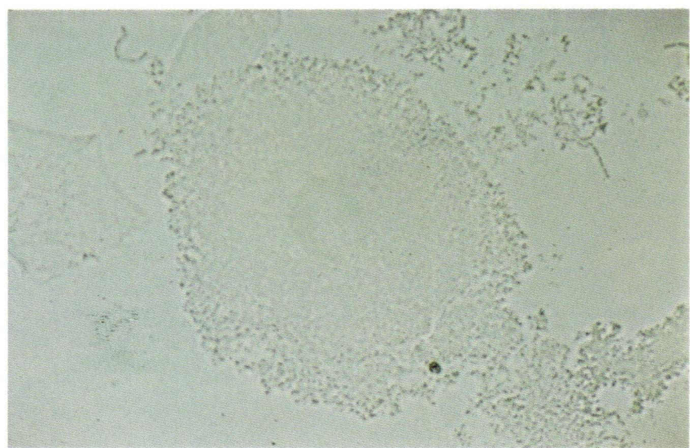

Fig 2–4. Squamous epithelial cell, showing degenerative changes. Notice granular cytoplasm and absence of clear delineation of either the nucleus or cytoplasmic margins (BF ×200).

plasmic margins may be nondistinct. Nonetheless, these alterations do not reflect a pathologic condition.

Squamous cells of the sediment originate in the lower end of the urinary tract (the distal third of both the male and female urethra) and the vagina. They may be present in small or large numbers, or may be absent from any given specimen. These cells, even when present in the sediment in large numbers, rarely have any pathologic significance. On occasion, however, the lower urinary tract may be involved by malignant change. When malignancy is present affecting the squamous epithelium (squamous carcinoma), the neoplastic epithelial cells are sloughed (exfoliated) into the urinary stream and often assume abnormal shapes and show nuclear abnormalities.[8, 45, 62, 64] In such instances the sediment should be treated as a cytologic specimen in the same manner as a fluid or secretion from any other organ, and stained by Papanicolaou techniques.

Squamous epithelial cells have a high refractive index and are easily observed with ordinary bright-field or interference microscopy (Figs 2–5 and 2–6). Because of their large size, small nuclei, and flattened shape, they ordinarily present no difficulties in recognition. Their presence is usually not recorded in routine urinalysis. However, if extremely large numbers are present, the observer may wish to record that fact. Squamous cells, like other cellular constituents, are counted as number per high-power microscopic field (no./hpf).

Transitional Epithelial Cells

Transitional epithelial cells (urothelial cells) originate in the transitional epithelium lining the renal pelvis and calyces, ureter, urinary bladder, and proximal two thirds of the urethra. Histologically, transitional epithelium is unique and easily recognized. It is distinguished from squamous epithelium because its cells have a polyhedral to spheric shape; measure approximately 20–30 μ in greatest diameter;

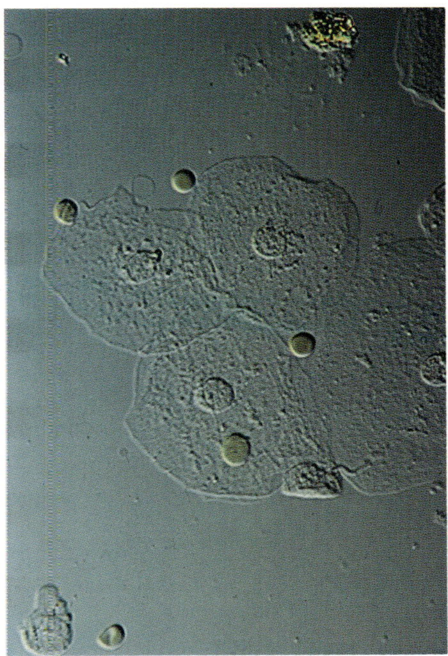

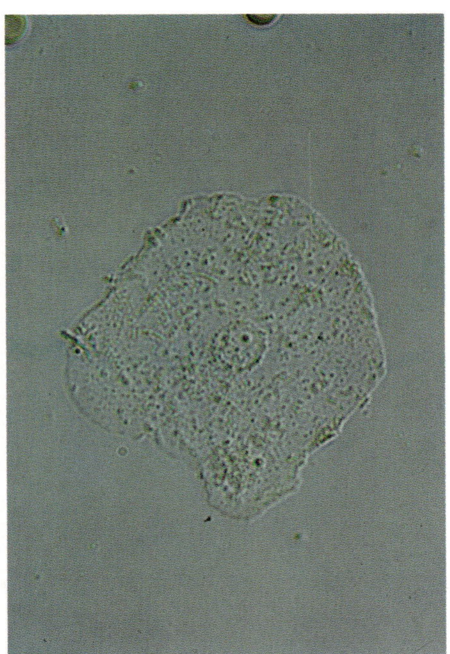

Fig 2–5 *(left).* Group of squamous epithelial cells with flattened shapes and granular cytoplasm. To compare relative sizes, note red blood cells. Red cells are approximately 7.5 μ in diameter (although they may be swollen on occasion), while squamous epithelial cell nuclei are approximately 7–12 μ in diameter. Granularity of the squamous cell cytoplasm and flattened shape of the cells are obvious (ICM ×160).

Fig 2–6 *(right).* Squamous epithelial cell in urine, characterized by spheric, central nucleus; flat shape; and granular or wrinkled cytoplasm (BF ×250).

and have relatively large, centrally placed, spheric nuclei (Fig 2–7). A distinctive physiologic characteristic of the transitional cell is that it readily accepts water. Therefore, those cells on the epithelial surface lining the lumen and in direct contact with the urine (ie, the cells sloughed into the urine and present in the sediment) are commonly observed as being spheric or "balloon-shaped" due to their enormous swelling.

Careful scrutiny of the sediment from a healthy person will usually reveal a few transitional cells. Their presence in small numbers is not pathologic and is to be expected. Large numbers of transitional cells are uncommon and usually denote an abnormal state. Instrumentation of the urinary tract may cause traumatic removal of these cells, in which case they may be observed in the sediment in sheets or groups.[53]

Once again, transitional epithelial cells are counted as number per high-power microscopic field (no./hpf). They may be differentially stained and distinguished with appropriate stains from similar-appearing cells that originate from epithelium lining the renal tubules (Fig 2–8).[57]

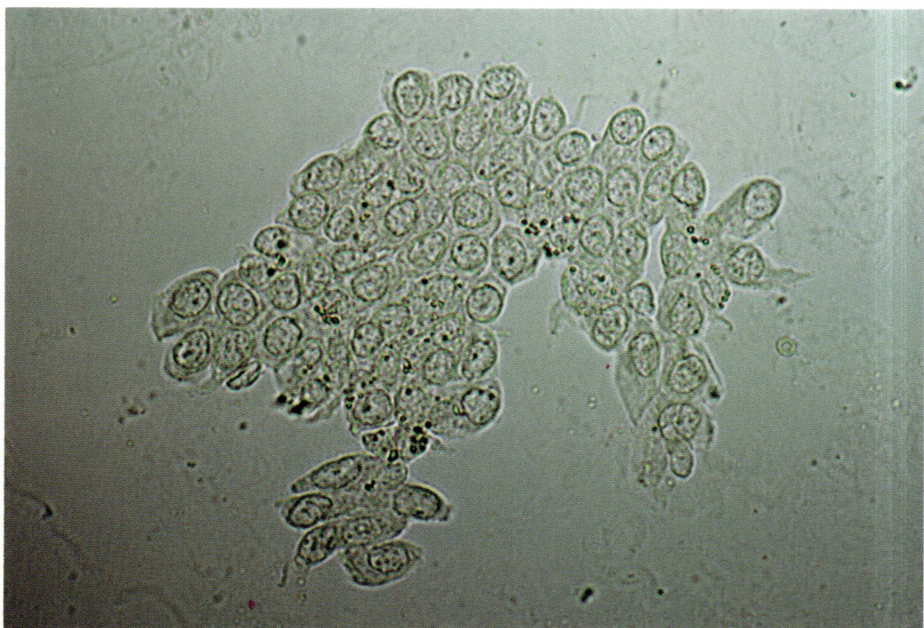

Fig 2–7. Group of transitional epithelial cells in urine, which are spheric and contain central, large nuclei (BF ×160).

Fig 2–8. Four transitional epithelial cells (center). Although there is much amorphous crystalline material in the field, the cells are still easily recognizable. Two are "tadpole"-shaped, whereas the other two are spheric (BF ×160).

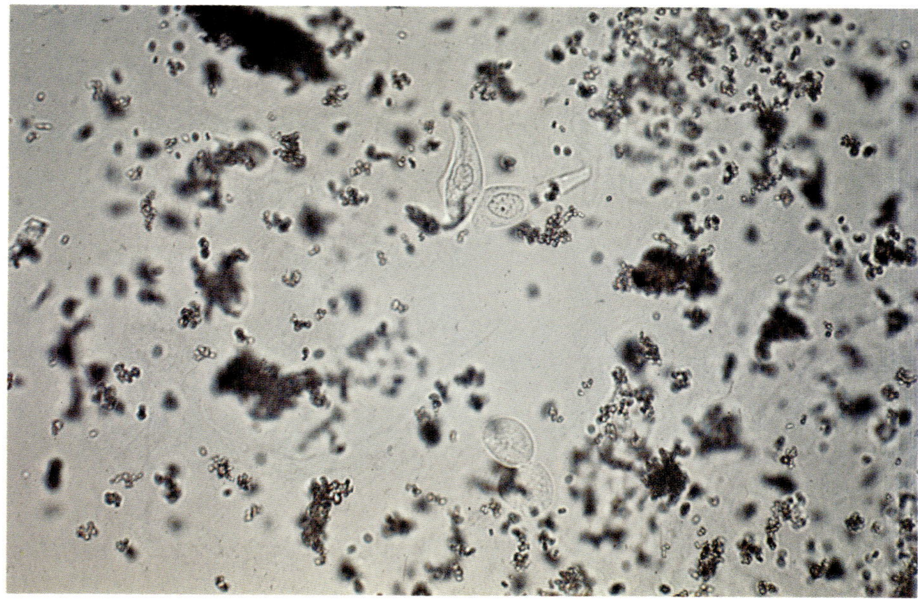

Transitional epithelial cells often occur in small groups, or *syncytia*, of several cells sloughing into the urine. However, more often they occur singly or in pairs and may be difficult to distinguish from renal epithelial cells, which have their origin in the kidney (Figs 2–9 and 2–10). In the normal sediment, unless markedly increased in number, transitional cells are usually not reported.

Another form of the transitional cell has been called a *decoy cell*.[13, 53] These are characterized by having red cytoplasm and large homogeneous blue or vacuolated curved nuclei when stained by the Sternheimer-Malbin technique. Decoy cells are associated with polyomavirus disease but may also be found in healthy persons.

Commonly, transitional epithelial neoplasms of the urinary tract exfoliate cells into the urine. These cells may be observed in the urinary sediment during routine analysis. Proper diagnosis can be made by ordinary cytologic techniques (Fig 2–11). The urinoscopist should suspect malignancies when large numbers of transitional cells appear in the urine and nuclear irregularities are present.

Fig 2–9 ***(left).*** Transitional epithelial cells, which are nearly spheric due to absorption of water and have large, central nuclei (BF ×320).

Fig 2–10 ***(right).*** Transitional epithelial cells in urinary sediment. This relief image clarifies spheric shape of these cells and nuclear detail and is superior to ordinary bright-field microscopy for this purpose (ICM ×320).

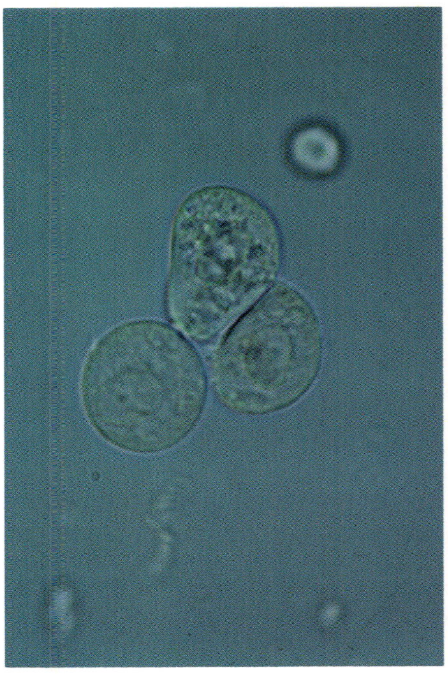

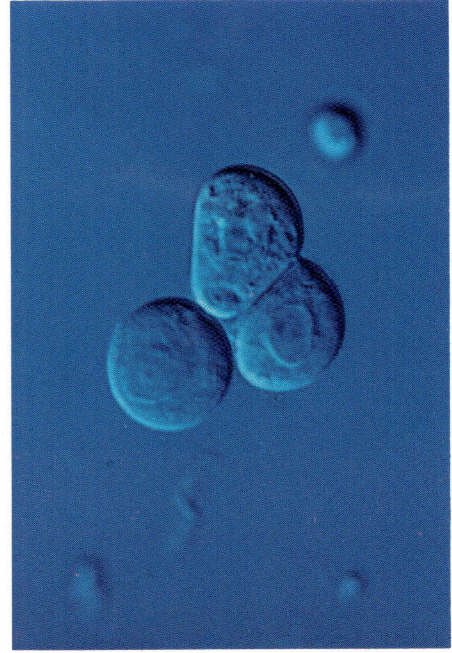

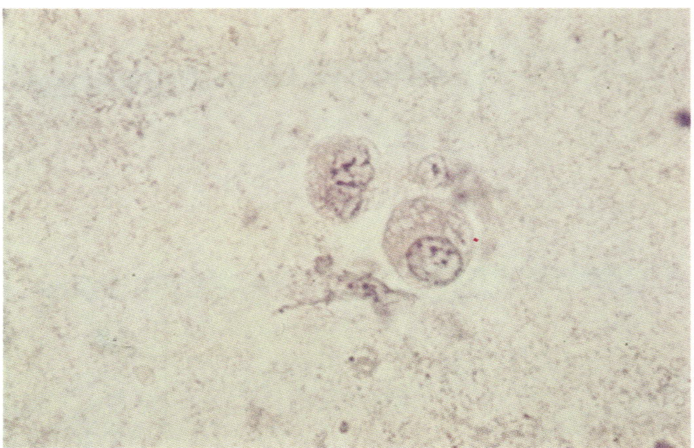

Fig 2–11. Malignant transitional epithelial cells observed during routine urinalysis. Nuclear hyperchromatism and irregularities are obvious (Pap stain ×250).

Renal Tubular Epithelial Cells

These cells are perhaps the most clinically important of all epithelial cells that occur in the urinary sediment. They derive their origin from epithelium lining the renal tubules. Diseases affecting the kidney in general, and the renal tubule specifically, may cause excess numbers of these cells to be sloughed into the sediment.[14]

Normal urinary sediment may contain small numbers of renal epithelial cells.[55] This is due to the fact that all epithelial cells undergo a constant process of regeneration, with a sloughing of the more mature or older cells, in this case into the urinary stream.

Renal tubular epithelial cells are difficult to distinguish from transitional epithelial cells in the urine. This is due to the fact that they are approximately the same size, 20 to 30 μ, and appear similar in their polyhedral shape and nuclear dimension. Histochemically, however, the differentiation may readily be made. In routine urinalysis, histochemical techniques are not ordinarily used, so the microscopist must pay careful attention to these cells when present. If the cells derive their origin from the proximal tubular epithelium of the nephron, they contain a microvillous border that can often be seen microscopically (Fig 2–12).[21] However, cells deriving their origin from the loop of Henle, distal tubule, or collecting duct do not have microvillous borders. Renal tubular epithelial cells when sloughed into the urine occur singly, but may also be seen in pairs. They have large, vesicular, central nuclei (Fig 2–13). The cells are polyhedral and do not swell as do transitional cells. Their nuclei may be eccentric and oriented towards one end of the cell. Renal epithelial cells are reported as number per high-power field, as are other epithelial cells.

When discussing the several varieties of renal epithelial cells in the urinary sediment, the question arises as to whether or not *intraglomerular cells* are found. Most probably they also slough into the urinary stream and are found in the urine.

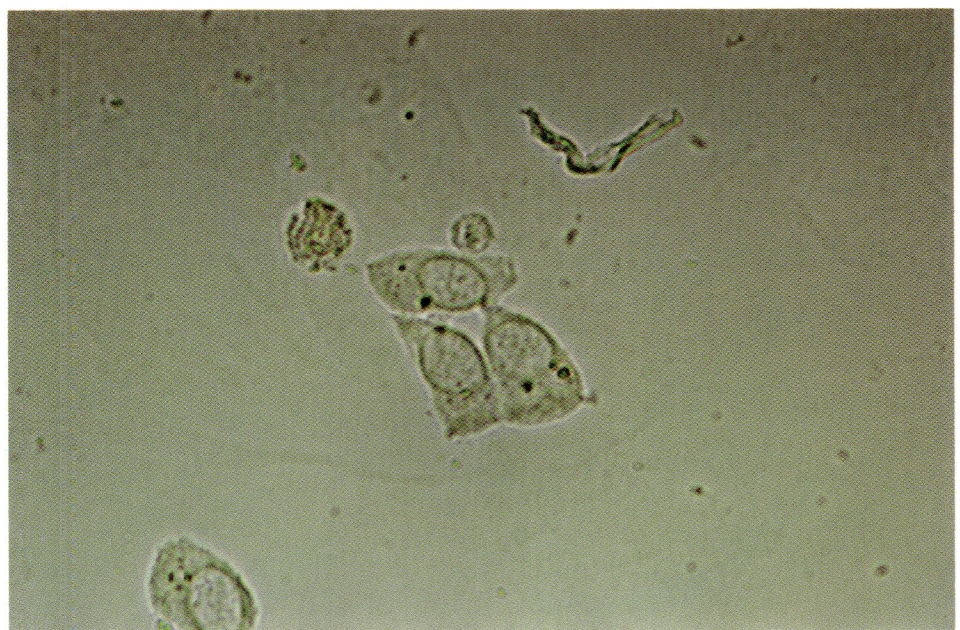

Fig 2–12. Three renal epithelial cells, whose nuclei are approximately the same size as an adjacent neutrophil. Renal epithelial cells are polyhedral and columnar. Their nuclei are often slightly off center and displaced towards the cell base. A microvillus border is evident in the cells shown here (BF ×200).

Fig 2–13. Group of attached renal tubular epithelial cells found in a case of acute glomerulonephritis. Background contains leukocytes and red blood cells. No microvillus border is present. Cytoplasm is somewhat granular, and nuclei are easily visualized (BF ×250).

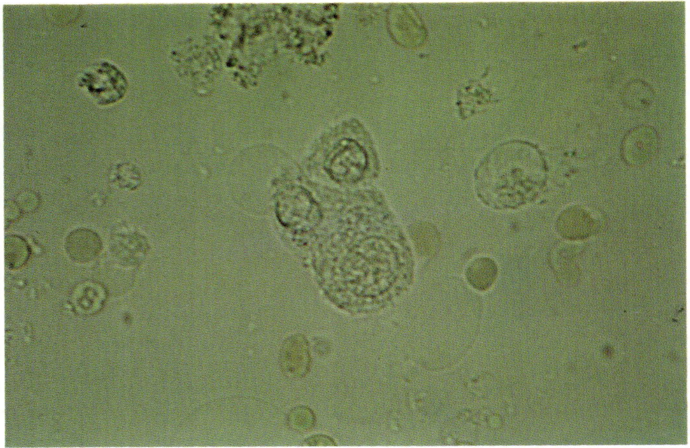

Unfortunately, with the present state of the art of urinoscopy, the methods employed to identify them specifically are inadequate. On a purely histologic basis, theoretically they may be *podocytes* (epithelial cells covering the glomerular capillary loops) or *parietal epithelial cells* (lining Bowman's space). The parietal epithelial cell embryologically has its origin from the same primordial cell as does the proximal tubular epithelium. However, in histologic preparations this cell appears flattened and similar to the squamous epithelial cells previously described. If the parietal epithelial cell does slough into the urinary stream, as is more than likely, its origin as a glomerular-lining cell may never be identified, since its morphologic characteristics are so similar to those of squamous epithelial cells that occur in the lower urinary tract or vagina.

Renal epithelial cells appear abnormally in the urine of patients with generalized viral diseases, especially cytomegalic inclusion disease (CID), measles, and viral hepatitis.[9, 10, 24] In such instances, the virus may secondarily involve the renal tubular epithelium and cause cell disruption and death. Especially in severe acute viral hepatitis, when the patient is jaundiced, tubular cells are sloughed in abundance and may be easily recognized in the urinary sediment due to their staining by bilirubin (Fig 2–14). In certain viral diseases, the presence of cytoplasmic inclusion bodies in sloughed renal tubular epithelial cells may be helpful in making a specific diagnosis. This is especially true in patients with CID involving the kidneys (Fig 2–15). Although cytologic examination of the urinary sediment is not ordinarily

Fig 2–14. Renal tubular epithelial cells with granular cytoplasm and eccentrically placed nuclei from a patient with viral hepatitis. Squamous cell (center) provides relative size comparison. Note that these renal tubular cells are yellow, indicating bile pigmentation (ICM ×160).

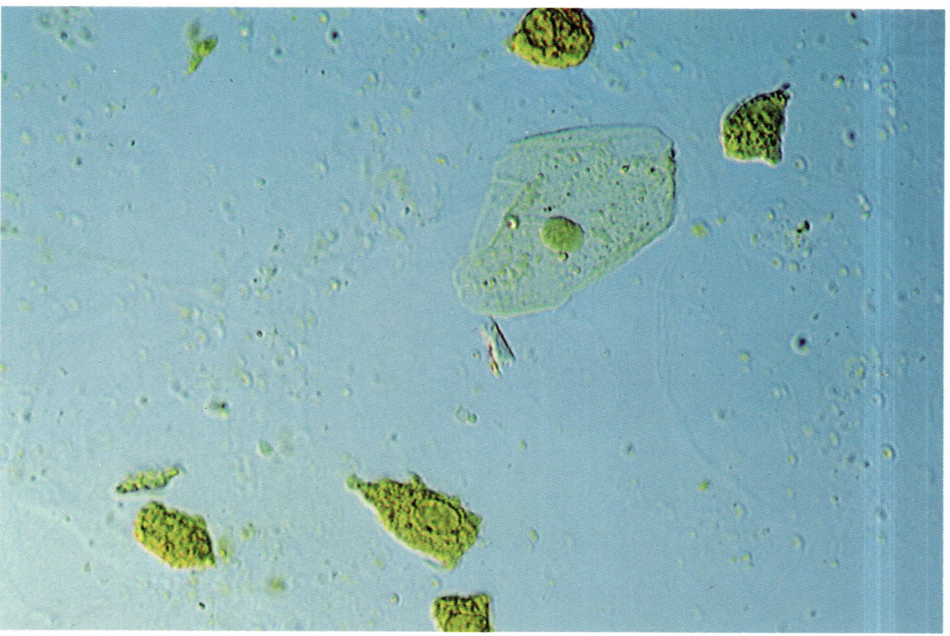

done on patients with measles, the virus may often involve the renal tubular epithelium; and when such involvement is present, many of the affected cells demonstrate typical measles inclusion bodies (Fig 2–16). In addition to generalized viral diseases, a host of toxins specifically affect the renal tubular epithelium. Classic examples of such toxicity are produced by a number of the ionized forms of heavy metals such as mercury, lead, uranium, and cadmium. Various agents used in cancer chemotherapy are also toxic to the renal tubular epithelium. Certain patients undergoing vigorous chemotherapy for cancer in which drugs such as methotrexate and 5-fluorouracil are used may have large numbers of renal tubular epithelial cells in the urinary sediment. Finally, other organic substances not ordinarily ingested by humans but used in suicide attempts or mistakenly taken by small children, such as diethylene glycol, cause severe renal tubular damage with the presence of large numbers of these cells in the urinary sediment (Fig 2–17).

Fig 2–15 ***(left).*** Renal tubular epithelial cells with cytoplasmic inclusion bodies, indicative of cytomegalic inclusion disease. Inclusion bodies are easily visible, as they are highly refractile, globular, and yellowish (BF ×320).

Fig 2–16 ***(right).*** Renal tubular epithelial cell with large, globular, red inclusion bodies, characteristic of measles virus (Giemsa stain ×630).

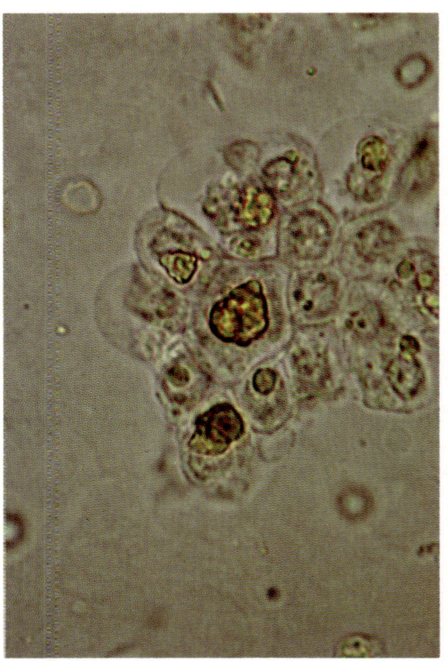

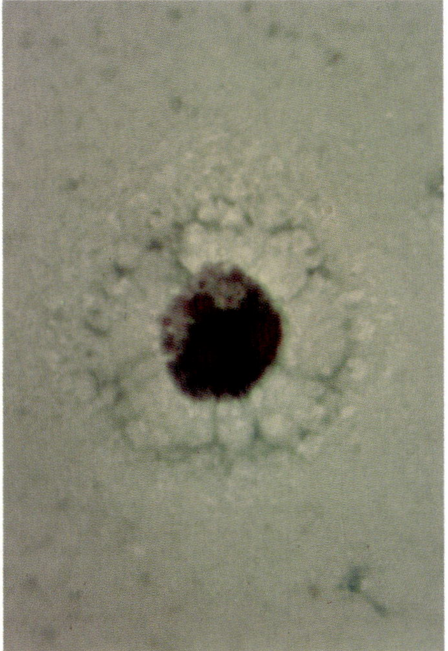

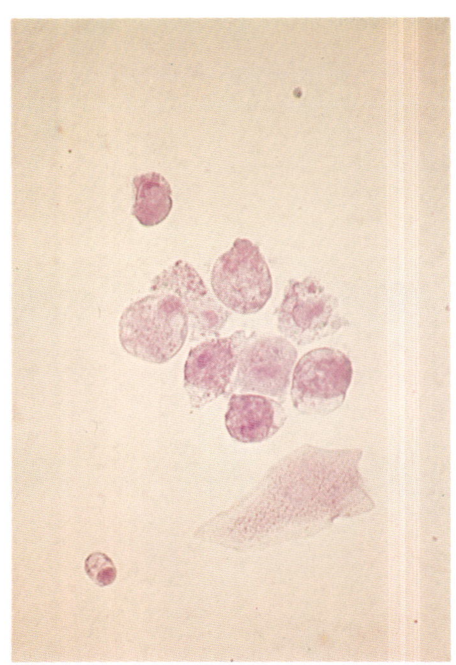

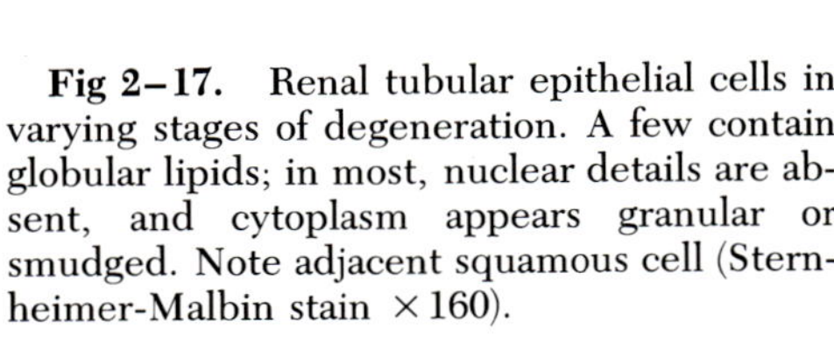

Fig 2–17. Renal tubular epithelial cells in varying stages of degeneration. A few contain globular lipids; in most, nuclear details are absent, and cytoplasm appears granular or smudged. Note adjacent squamous cell (Sternheimer-Malbin stain ×160).

Oval Fat Bodies and Lipiduria

Fat in the urine is called *lipiduria* and is a pathologic finding that ordinarily indicates a relatively severe type of renal dysfunction. Fat is found in the urine either intracellularly (oval fat bodies), as free fat globules (neutral lipid), or incorporated into urinary casts (fatty casts).[20, 25] Fatty casts will be discussed in Chapter 6.

In a wide variety of disease states, as well as in renal transplant patients, increased numbers of renal tubular epithelial cells may be found in the urinary sediment.[5, 9, 24, 33] They are often increased in patients in whom specific toxins, viruses, and various bodily metabolic products affect the renal tubules directly. Ordinarily these cells are not difficult to recognize, and except for some degenerative changes such as a vacuolar cytoplasm and nuclear disruption, they appear no different from the normal tubular epithelial cells described previously. However, they often are observed to have severe intracellular degenerative changes that indicate a specific disease process affecting the tubular portion of the nephron, causing the cells to die and be sloughed into the urinary stream. As tubular epithelial cells degenerate, the lipid in their cytoplasm may become microscopically visible, whereas in the normal cell it is not (Fig 2–18). In addition, in many renal diseases various lipids (especially cholesterol), which may be present in high concentration in the glomerular filtrate, are absorbed by these tubular epithelial cells and are recognizable as spheric, globular, yellowish tan vacuoles in the cytoplasm. When these same cells are viewed with the polarizing microscope, these intracytoplasmic globular bodies are perceived as being doubly refractile or birefringent, and display a symmetric "Maltese-cross" pattern (Figs 2–19 and 2–20).[25] Fat bodies have the propensity for absorbing sudanophilic dyes. When stained with these dyes, they appear as orange spheres under ordinary bright-field microscopy (Fig 2–21). In rare instances, an occasional oval fat body may be observed in the urine of a supposedly healthy subject. However, since it is well known that abnormalities of the urinary sediment may precede overt disease, especially viral diseases that affect the kidney, the finding of any renal tubular epithelial cells in the urine with visible lipids in their cytoplasm must be considered pathologic.

Free fat may be present in the urine in certain conditions; it bears mention here since it is ordinarily associated with oval fat bodies. Globules of free fat characteristically appear in the sediment as light yellowish brown spherules that vary greatly in size. Some may be miniscule (2–4 μ), while others may be as large as renal epithelial cells (20 μ). This neutral fat can be stained with Sudan III and IV dyes but is most easily recognized (as is intracellular lipid) by means of polarized light, since these lipids also have the property of anisotropism. Lipid birefringence may be distinguished from other anisotropic "cross" patterns, such as that seen with talcum granules.

Globular lipids are found in the urine in a wide variety of clinical conditions. Among the most common of these is the *nephrotic syndrome*, a clinical syndrome consisting of lipiduria, lipidemia, hypercholesterolemia, and edema. Specific diseases in which this free form of lipid is frequently present in the urine are advanced diabetes mellitus, lipoid nephrosis, and toxic renal tubular nephrosis.

Fig 2–18. Three oval fat bodies (renal epithelial cells) in which cytoplasmic lipids are present as highly refractile spheric globules. Nucleus of cell (lower right) is still clearly visible (BF ×160).

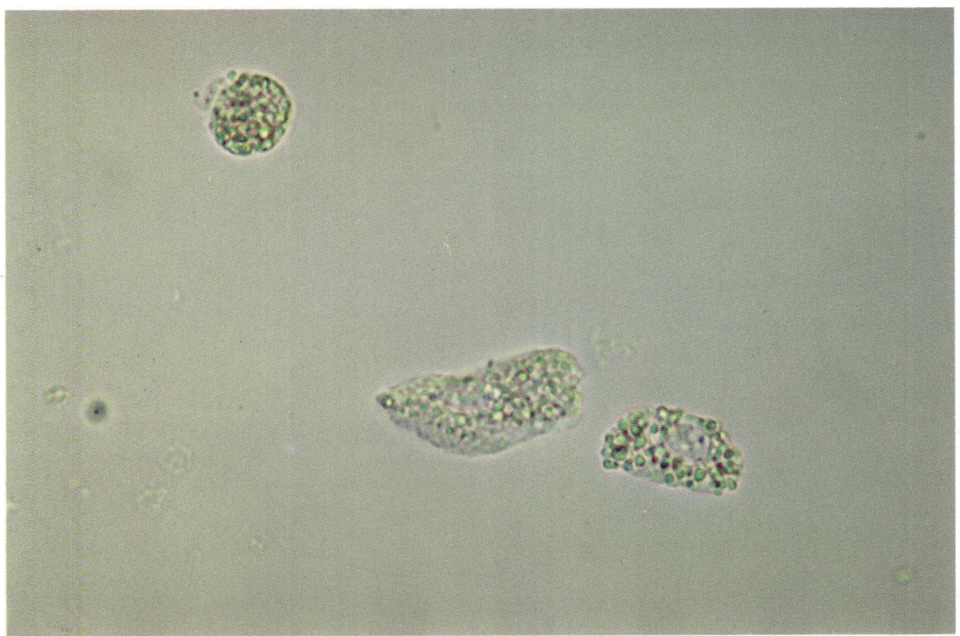

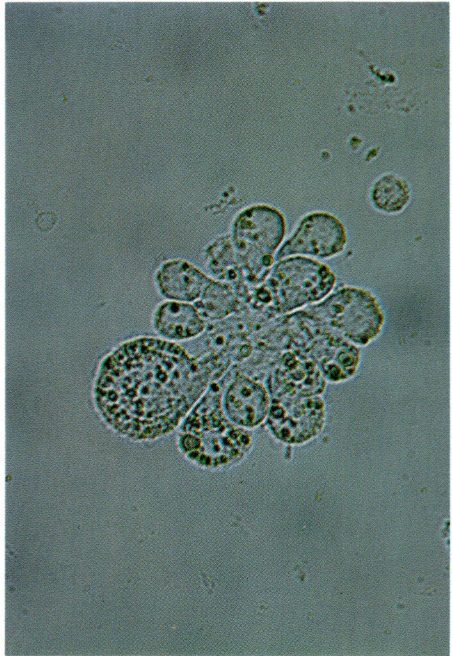

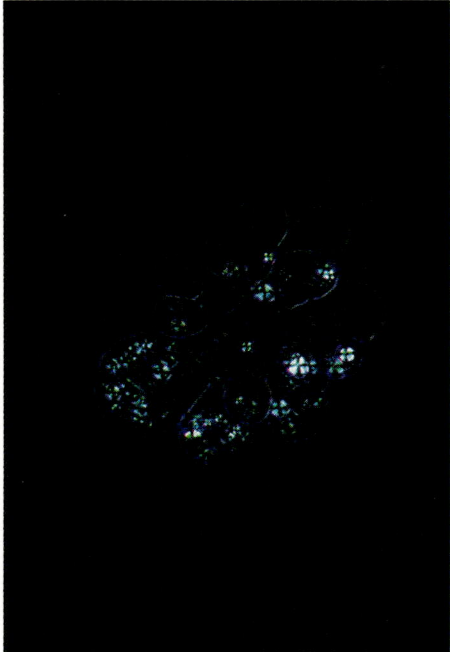

Fig 2–19 ***(left).*** Group of oval fat bodies. The lipid globules in a contiguous group of renal tubular epithelial cells are highly refractile, of varying size, and easily seen. The cells have obviously undergone considerable degeneration, and nuclear characteristics are not apparent (BF ×200).

Fig 2–20 ***(right).*** Oval fat bodies. Same group of renal tubular epithelial cells was shown in Figure 2–19. "Maltese-cross" patterns are readily observed and demonstrate birefringence of cytoplasmic lipids in these degenerating cells (Pol ×160).

Other Epithelial Cells

Several other varieties of polyhedral cuboidal to columnar epithelial cells may infrequently be found in the urinary sediment.[53] These cells derive their origin from the prostate gland, paraurethral glands, and seminal vesicle. They may occur singly or in clumps and may be impossible to differentiate from renal tubular epithelial cells without the aid of histochemical stains.

Corpora amylacea, a type of calculi produced by the epithelium lining the prostatic glands, may occasionally be observed in the sediment, often in association with prostatic epithelial cells. These spheric, laminated, calcific bodies are easily identified by their characteristic appearance and eosinophilic staining characteristics (see Fig 9–1).

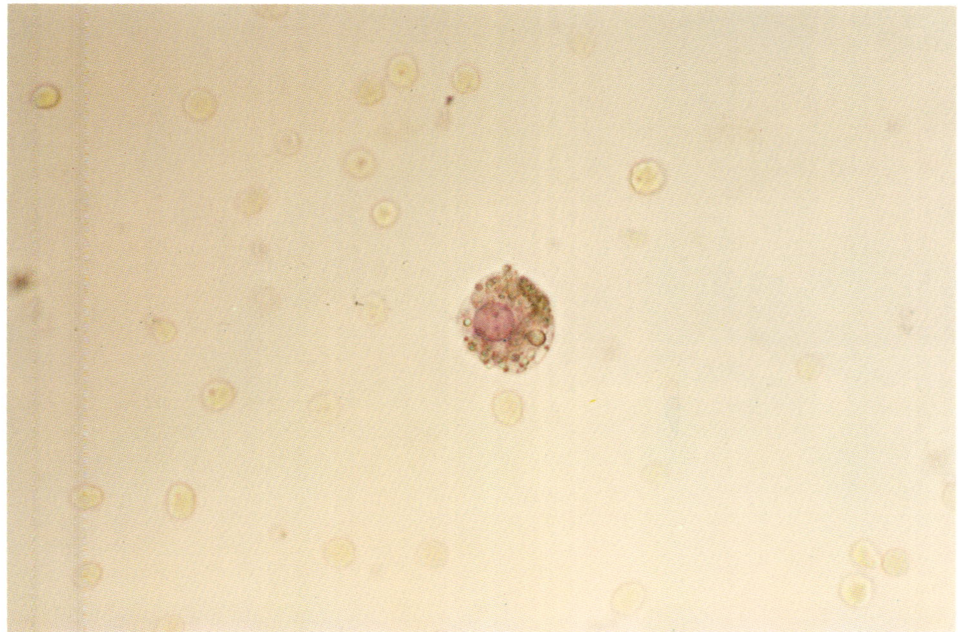

Fig 2–21. Degenerating renal tubular epithelial cell with visible cytoplasmic lipid (oval fat body) and red nucleus. Red blood cells are present in the background (Sternheimer-Malbin stain ×160).

BLOOD CELLS

Peripheral blood cells are normally present in the urinary sediment,[1, 3] though in small numbers. The most frequently occurring cells, and also the most easily recognized, are polymorphonuclear neutrophils (PMNs) and erythrocytes (RBCs) (Fig 2–22).[34, 38] In addition, platelets may be observed when the urine is carefully scrutinized (using the sophisticated techniques of electron microscopy).[59] Besides PMNs, other leukocytes may be present.[38] These "other" leukocytes are found infrequently in healthy persons, but are observed in certain disease states in which the peripheral circulation contains large numbers of them or in certain pathologic conditions affecting the kidney or lower urinary tract.[29, 48]

White Blood Cells

Under normal conditions, the polymorphonuclear neutrophil is the white blood cell most frequently found in the urinary sediment. This cell is identified with ease and should not be confused with other cells of similar size (ie, renal epithelial cells).[38] Recognition of the PMN is facilitated by knowing that it has a multilobed nucleus (segmented nucleus) and granular cytoplasm. The cell ordinarily measures 12–15 μ in greatest diameter. Staining the urinary sediment by the Wright's or Giemsa techniques often helps in identification of these cells but is ordinarily not necessary for specific identification (Fig 2–23).

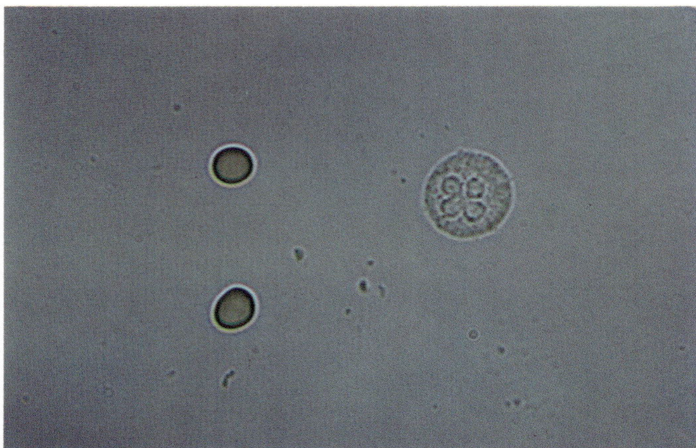

Fig 2–22. Neutrophil and two erythrocytes in urinary sediment. The WBC with granular cytoplasm and multilobate nucleus is approximately twice as large as the RBCs (BF ×250).

Fig 2–23. Large number of neutrophils, many revealing multilobed nuclei, characteristic of this cell type (Sternheimer-Malbin stain ×250).

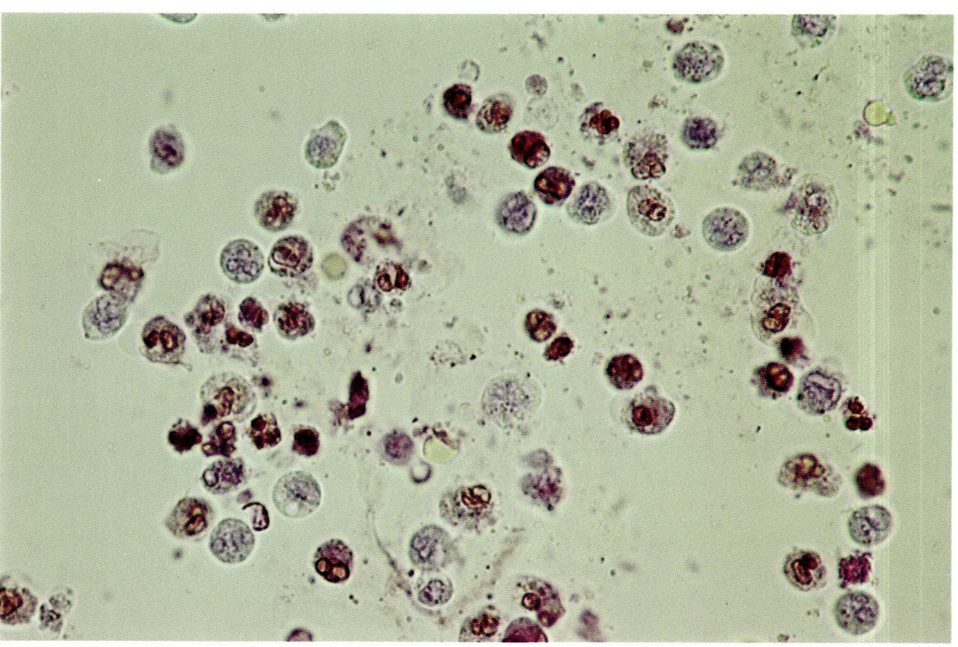

Lymphocytes or monocytes are infrequently observed in the normal urine. They are difficult to identify with accuracy unless special smears are made or cytocentrifugation techniques[53] applied and appropriate stains used (Wright's or Giemsa stains). When this is done, however, a rare lymphocyte or monocyte may be seen in the normal sediment.

In the normal sediment, the number of PMNs present per high-power microscopic field is usually 3–5.[21] Increases above this range ordinarily indicate inflammatory conditions involving the kidney or lower urinary tract.[32] Disease states of an inflammatory nature may be monitored semiquantitatively by simply counting the number of these cells present in a constant volume of concentrated urine at regular intervals. Ameboid motion of leukocytes in the urine is an interesting feature and may be observed provided the urine is fresh and the observer is patient (Fig 2–24). Ameboid motion is much more frequently seen in conjunction with bacteriuria. In such instances phagocytosis of the microorganisms is a common feature but is often unrecognized unless the observer is specifically looking for it (Figs 2–25 and 2–26).

Fig 2–24. Leukocytes in urine showing ameboid motion. Cell in the center has a pseudopod extending from its cytoplasm (ICM ×160).

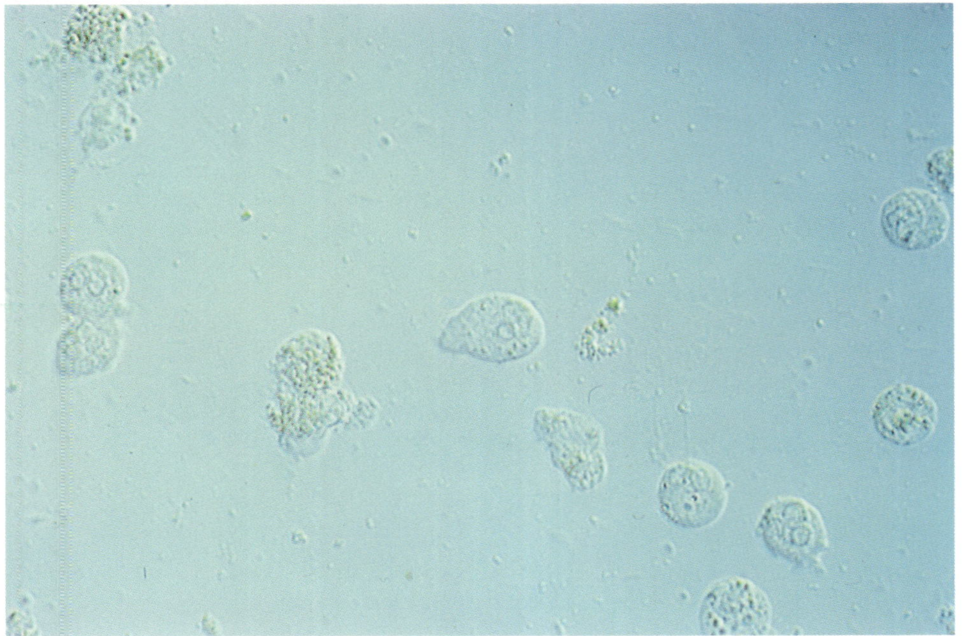

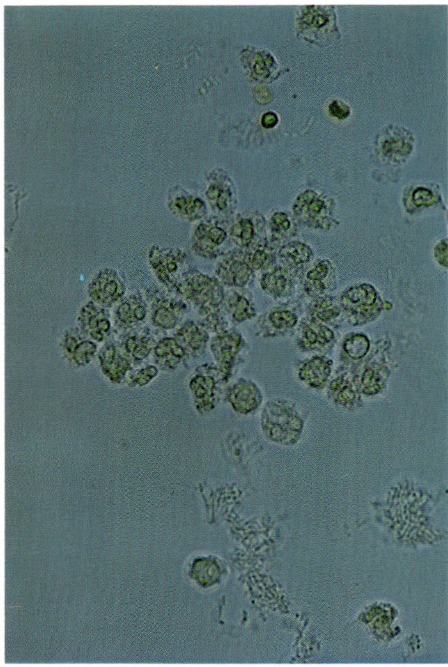

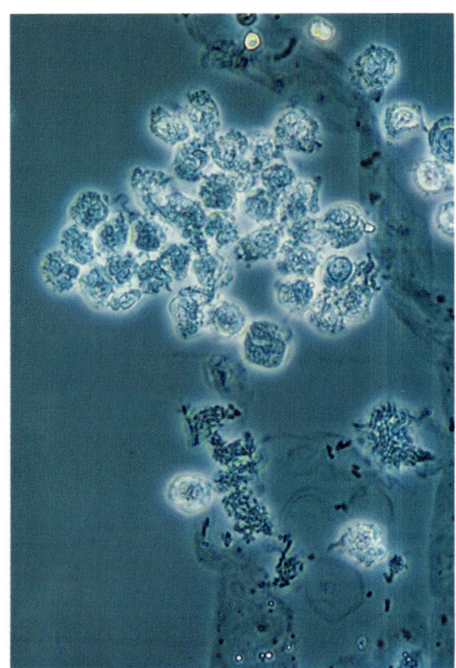

Fig 2–25 ***(left).*** Numerous PMNs and bacteria. A few mononuclear leukocytes accompany this exudate (BF ×200).

Fig 2–26 ***(right).*** Same field as that in Figure 2–25, but taken by phase-contrast microscopy. Note that the cells are readily visible, and bacteria are especially prominent as black rods. There is also a scattering of mucus fibrils (PH ×200).

Red Blood Cells

Erythrocytes are normally present in the urine in small numbers (0–3 per high-power field) (see Fig 2–22).[34] Depending on the osmotic gradient of the urine that surrounds these cells, they may be swollen, of normal size, or crenated.[21] For crenation to occur, the red cells must be present in a hypertonic milieu. Since the red cell membrane is permeable to various solutes in the urine, as well as to water, changes in size and shape of the red cell are commonplace (Figs 2–27 and 2–28). Increased numbers of red blood cells (RBCs) in the urine *(hematuria)* are pathologic and usually indicate disease in the kidney or lower urinary tract.[31, 44]

Red cells are perhaps the easiest of all cells to identify in the urinary sediment. The reason is that they are of relatively consistent size, have a biconcave disc shape, and are pigmented with hemoglobin (Fig 2–29). Their normal diameter of 7.5 μ is useful in making size comparisons when surveying other cells and sediment elements.

The hemoglobin molecule is the major component of the red blood cell, and if lysis of these cells occurs when they are present in abnormally large numbers, hemoglobinuria may be detected by dipstick methodology or chemical means.[16] However, when small numbers of RBCs are present, as in healthy persons, ordinary dipstick methods are not sensitive enough to detect their presence.

Fig 2–27. Red blood cells in urine (BF ×160).

Fig 2–28. Many crenated RBCs in urinary sediment. Although they show hemoglobin pigmentation and are of uniform size, their biconcavity is more difficult to discern (BF ×250).

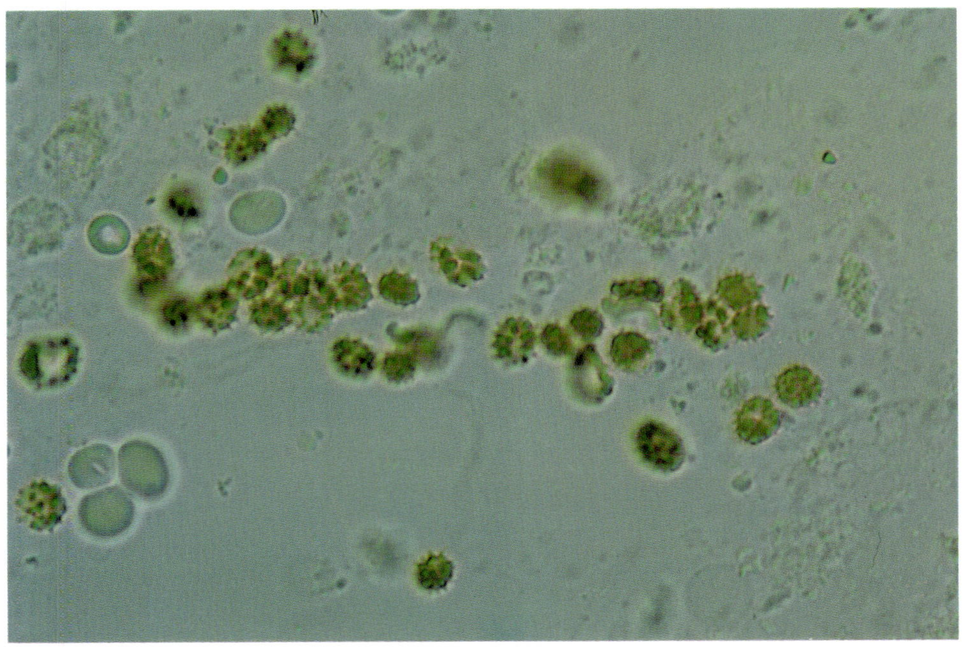

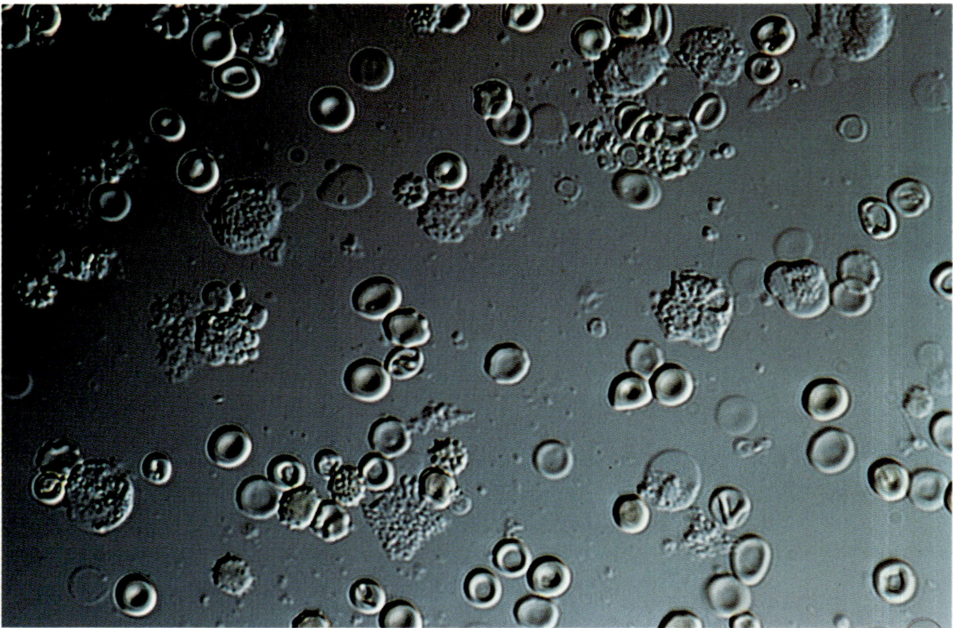

Fig 2–29. Red and white blood cells in urine. Under ICM, their morphologic characteristics are more obvious. Biconcavity, hemoglobin pigmentation, and regular size of the red cells are apparent. In some leukocytes, multilobate nuclei and granular cytoplasm are pronounced (ICM ×250).

SPERMATOZOA

Spermatozoa may be motile or nonmotile in urine (Fig 2–30). Motility depends on time of ejaculation in reference to the performance of urinalysis. Urine itself is toxic to spermatozoa, and absence of motility may simply be a factor of how long the urine has been allowed to stand prior to examination. Abnormal morphologic forms of spermatozoa (Fig 2–31) are observed with no greater frequency in the urine than in seminal fluid when these examinations are done separately and promptly. Abnormal spermatozoa are rarely seen in normal subjects, but if sterility is a clinical problem, they should be reported. In many instances, early dissolution and lysis of sperm forms are observed in the urine by noting that many of the spermatozoa have no tails—again, a fact crudely related to how long the specimen has remained unexamined. Spermatozoa may be found in either male or female urine, and their numbers vary greatly.

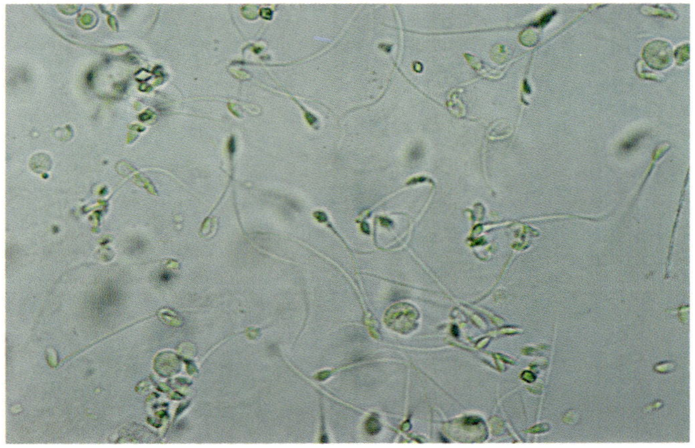

Fig 2–30. Large number of spermatozoa in urine (BF ×200).
Fig 2–31. Abnormal, two-headed sperm in urinary sediment (Sternheimer-Malbin stain ×320).

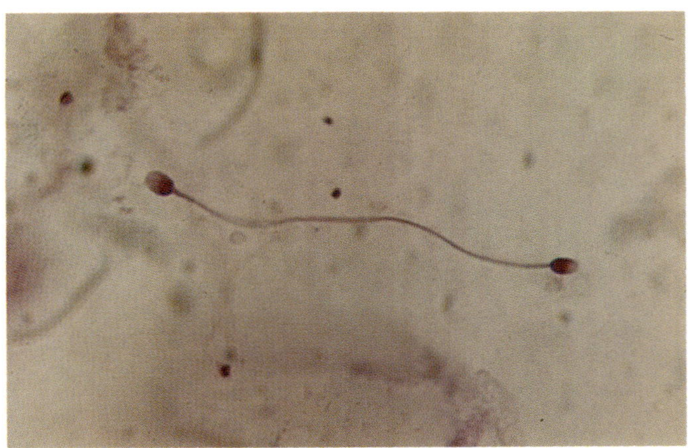

ADDIS COUNT

The Addis count is a quantitative method for determining the number of formed elements present in the urinary sediment over a prolonged period of time, ie, 12 hours.[3] Although no longer in common clinical use, this method does provide a means of following the course of an active renal disease.[1] The urine is collected in a glass jug or plastic bag over a 12-hour period; fluids, but not food, are restricted during the collection interval. The total volume of urine is measured, a 10-ml aliquot is centrifuged, and 9 ml of supernatant is discarded. The remaining urine, which includes the sediment, is then mixed thoroughly; and a sample is placed in a Neubauer counting chamber. Using a low-power (10×) objective, the number of cells and casts is counted in the chamber's nine large squares, each square representing 0.0001 ml of urine. Finally, by means of a relatively simple calculation, a quantitative estimation of the number of sediment elements per milliliter of urine over the 12-hour collection period is obtained.

There are several reasons why the Addis count is no longer used routinely to assess the course and predict the prognosis of an active renal disease. The technique is time consuming, laborious, and fraught with inaccuracies. A major problem is that many of the sediment elements disintegrate during the 12-hour collection period. Also, there are more efficient semiquantitative methods for analyzing sediment that are available today; their clinical applications provide comparable results to the Addis count, yet are more cost effective. In these methods, a predetermined volume of urine is centrifuged, and the elements are counted in a chamber of standard volume (see Chapter 10).

From a historic viewpoint, one of the main contributions of the Addis count was recognition of the fact that the healthy person excreted relatively large numbers of cells and casts in the urine. For instance, under normal circumstances in a routine urinalysis, one would expect to find an occasional hyaline cast, one or two erythrocytes, and two to three leukocytes per high-power microscopic field. The Addis count demonstrated that the actual number of casts in the healthy person's urine may be 6,000 every 12 hours; and the erythrocytes and leukocytes may number as many as 500,000 and 1,000,000, respectively, over the same time interval. Obviously, in the disease state, these numbers may increase markedly.

3. BACTERIA AND FUNGI

Normally, the urine is free of microorganisms. However, since it is ordinarily collected under nonsterile conditions and is an excellent culture medium, bacteria and yeasts are commonly found in what is otherwise considered "normal" urine (Figs 3–1 and 3–2). The fact that bacteria are or are not present in any given urine sediment is not nearly as important as whether or not the microorganisms are accompanied by inflammatory cells and measurable amounts of protein.[21, 44]

Fig 3–1 ***(left).*** Squamous cells and bacteria in urine. Bacillary forms are seen in chains or singly. Squamous cells are included in the field for size comparison (BF ×250).

Fig 3–2 ***(right).*** Same field as shown in Figure 3–1, but with phase-contrast technique, which enables bacterial forms to be seen easily. Note that no leukocytes are present—a finding associated with bacterial contamination of the urine rather than a urinary tract infection (PH ×250).

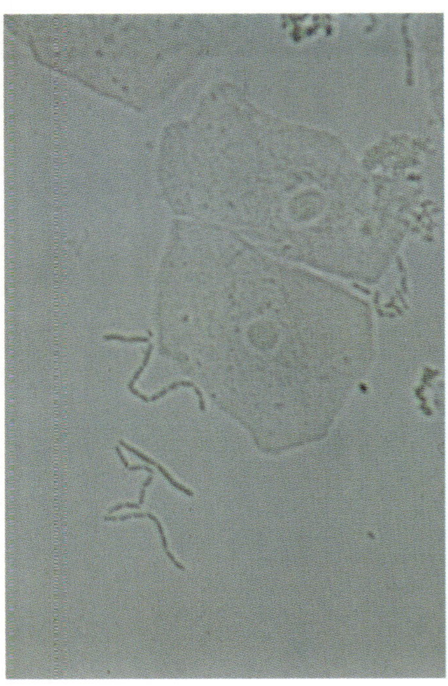

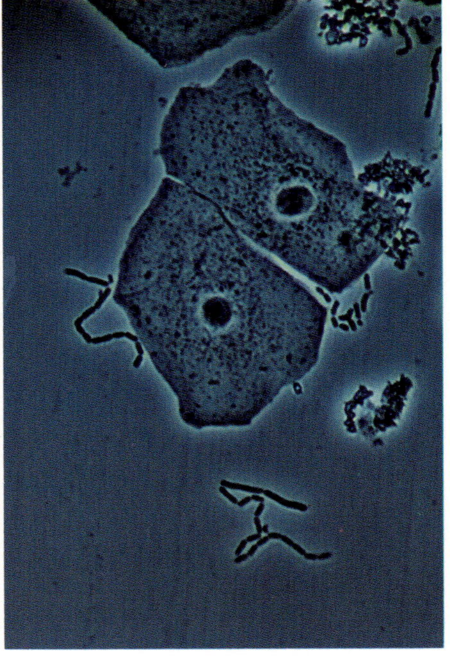

Contamination of the urine by bacteria or fungi may occur through the following mechanisms:

(1) Contamination of the vagina or lower urinary tract. (To help avoid this, it is important to use a "clean-catch" technique of urine specimen collection.)
(2) Contamination of collection cups, centrifuge tubes, jars, and bottles.
(3) Airborne contamination when urine is allowed to sit unrefrigerated and exposed to the air.

When bacteria are observed in urine, a decision must be made as to whether they are pathogenic or not. This is usually done by means of microscopic observation. One must know whether the bacteria are present in conjunction with inflammatory cells, usually large numbers of PMNs (Fig 3–3). In the absence of inflammatory cells, bacteria in the urine are more than likely contaminants and are therefore probably not pathogens. However, they may be present in large numbers. This may give a positive protein and nitrite test result when chemical examination of the urine is performed and may produce a cloudy appearance when observed macroscopically. Colony counts of more than 100,000 and a urine culture are of considerable help in distinguishing contaminant bacteriuria from pathologic bacteriuria, provided, of course, that the determination is made on freshly collected urine.[27]

Recently, an immunologic means of distinguishing upper- from lower-urinary-tract infection has been developed, the antibody-coated bacteria (ACB) test. Based

Fig 3–3. Low-power view of bacteria in urine with several leukocytes in the field. Bacteria are bacillary and diffusely scattered throughout (Sternheimer-Malbin stain ×100).

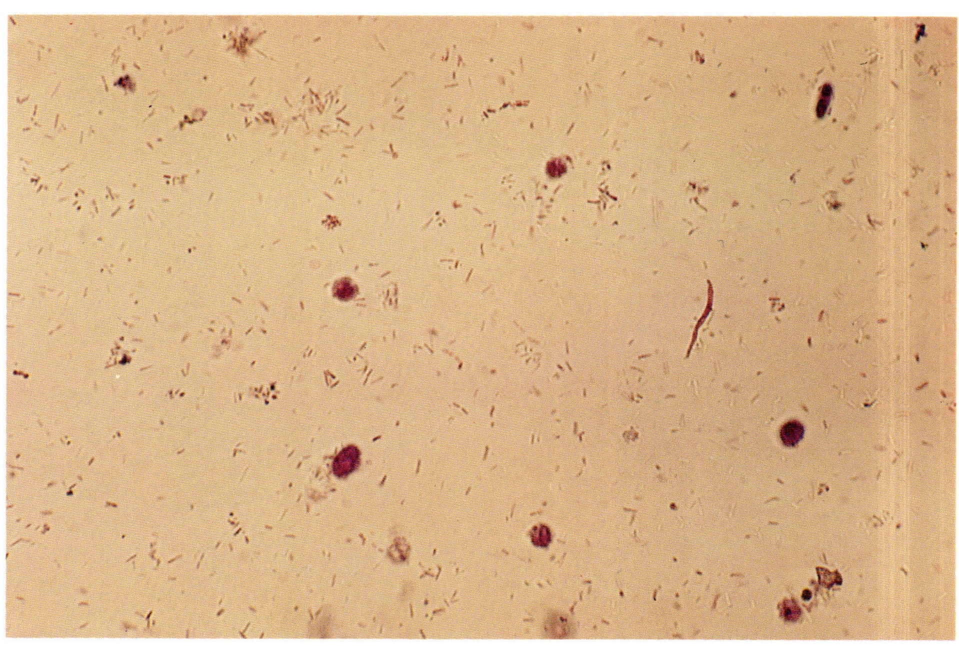

on the fact that the kidney coats infecting bacteria with protein and the lower urinary tract epithelium does not, this immunologic test, while not foolproof, assists in distinguishing intrarenal infections from those involving the lower urinary tract.[47]

Morphologically, bacteria assume either bacillary or coccal forms (see Figs 3–1 and 3–2). They may stain either gram-positive or gram-negative, and, if considered pathogenic, should be cultured for accurate identification. The most common contaminants in the urine are gram-negative bacilli, most often *Escherichia coli*.

Fungi are also observed as contaminants of the urine with great frequency (Fig 3–4). However, fungi are more likely to be pathogenic than bacteria. This is especially true in patients having certain metabolic diseases such as diabetes mellitus. Fungi are morphologically easier to recognize than bacteria because of their generally larger size, relatively thick walls, and rapid dividing times so that they occur in clumps (Fig 3–5). Budding and hyphal forms are also commonly observed, especially when the urine is allowed to remain for long periods of time at room temperature (Fig 3–6). Again, if there is no inflammatory exudate, the observed fungi are probably contaminants rather than pathogens.

Yeast microorganisms may be easily confused with red blood cells or fat globules. Therefore, careful scrutiny should be made of any spheric particle in the urine to determine its exact origin.

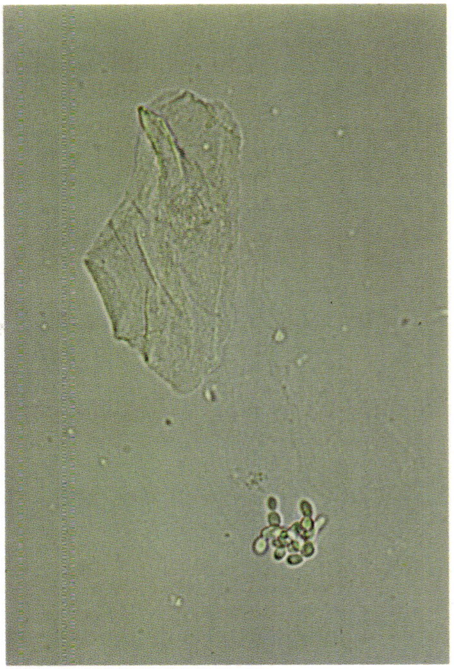

Fig 3–4. Budding yeast in urine. Squamous epithelial cell is included for size comparison. Note that PMNs are not seen. This suggests that the yeasts are contaminants and unrelated to a urinary tract infection (BF ×200).

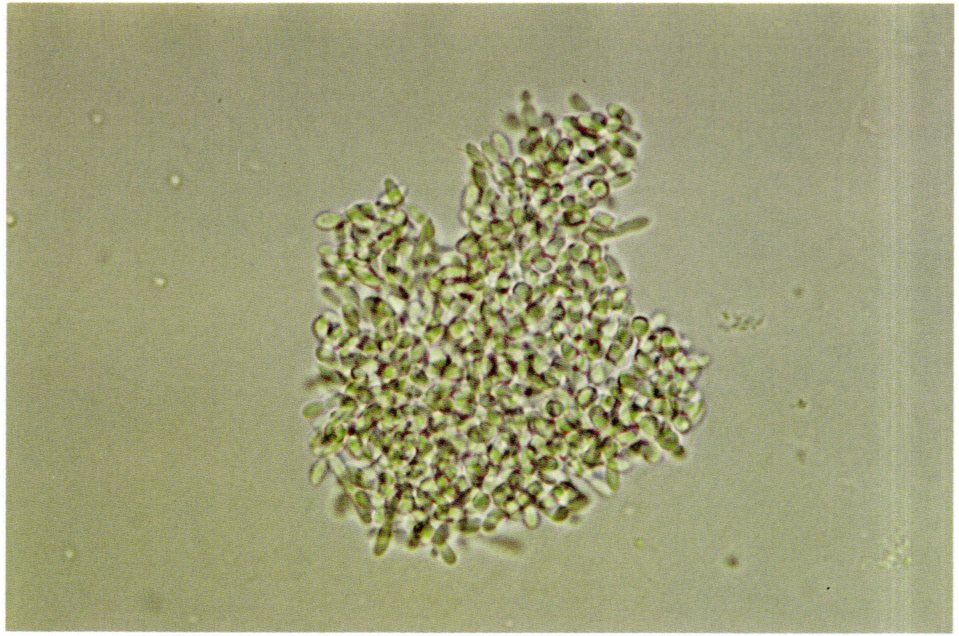

Fig 3–5. Clump of budding yeast forms, which occur as single spherules or in groups, as shown here (BF ×200).

Fig 3–6. Branching yeasts with hyphal forms. There are several accompanying PMNs, indicating a urinary tract infection (ICM ×160).

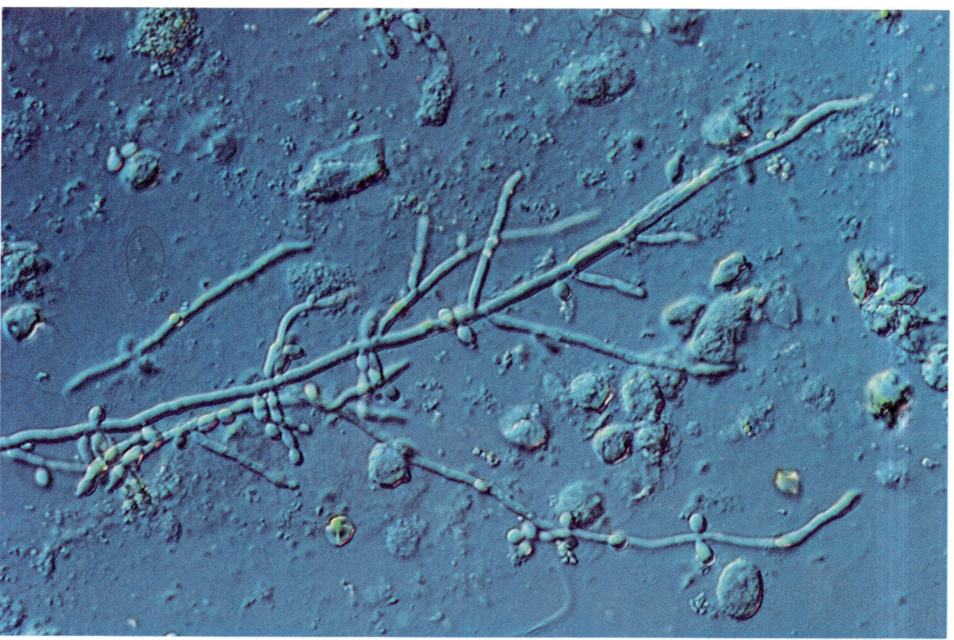

4. MUCUS

Mucus abounds in the human urinary sediment. It is seen more frequently in the urine of women but is also present in urine from men. It is formed by the cells of the glands lining the lower genitourinary tract and is also produced by the vaginal epithelium. The presence or absence of mucus in the urinary sediment has no pathologic significance. However, its recognition is of importance in that the uninitiated observer may inadvertently confuse it with pathologic urinary sediment elements.

Morphologically, mucus strands are recognized without undue difficulty.[39] They have a very low refractive index and may be missed by ordinary bright-field microscopy (Figs 4–1 and 4–2). However, when the microscope condenser is sufficiently lowered and the iris diaphragm stopped down, the thin fibrillar strands of urinary mucus are observed. These strands take a variety of forms and shape, but most are delicate and threadlike and are tortuous or serpentine. Mucus occurs indiscriminately throughout the microscopic field.

Mucus may easily be mistaken for hyaline casts. It is therefore incumbent on the observer to distinguish mucus from other formed elements of the sediment.[21] Mucus has approximately the same refractive index as hyaline casts, but it does not have the typical smooth parallel sides, cylindrical shape, and appropriate size.

Mucus strands are easily observed when phase-contrast or interference-contrast microscopy is used in examination of the sediment.[20] With phase-contrast microscopy, mucus strands are recognized as being fibrillar, thin, wavy, and of low refractive index (Figs 4–3 and 4–4). Interference-contrast microscopy shows mucus as three-dimensional, thin, wavy strands of semisolid mucopolysaccharide material arranged in haphazard fashion and assuming no particular morphologic shape or characteristics.[19] Size comparisons are important in distinguishing mucus threads from hyaline casts.

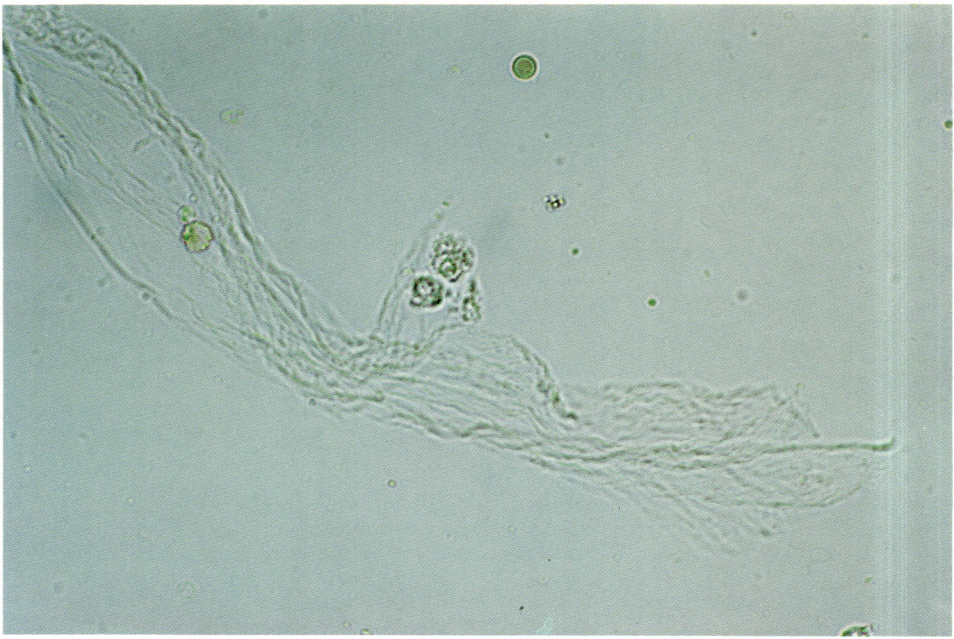

Fig 4–1. Mucus, especially visible in the center. Two entrapped white cells and two erythrocytes are also present. Mucus strands are fibrillar and delicate and have a very low refractive index (BF ×160).

Fig 4–2. Mucus threads in urine, which are easily seen here. Note their structural detail. This is the same field as shown in Figure 4–1 (PH ×160).

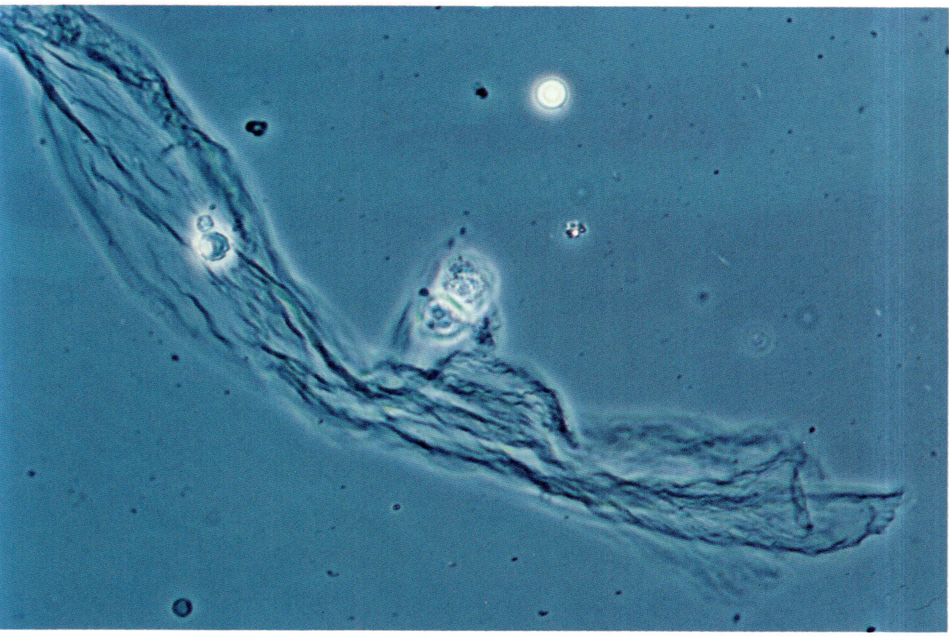

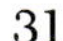

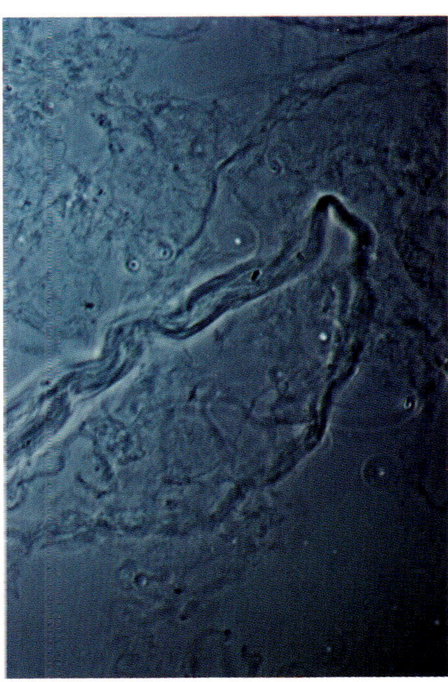

Fig 4–3. Dense accumulation of mucus strands. Those in the center simulate a hyaline cast. However, on close inspection, the filamentous threads do not actually form a solid structure, ie, a cast. Many other mucus filaments are present in the background (PH ×160).

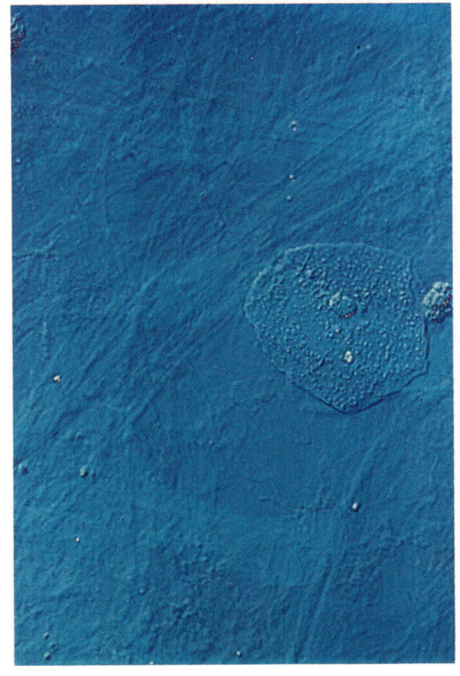

Fig 4–4. Mucus filaments, superimposed upon one another. They are easily defined, structureless, fibrillar material of low density. For size comparison, note squamous epithelial cell (ICM ×160).

5. CRYSTALLURIA

Anne Thompson, MT (ASCP), SH

Crystals are commonly found in human urinary sediment. It is fundamentally important for the observer to identify the crystals that are normally present in the urine and to distinguish them from abnormal crystals, which are associated with various disease states and are not ordinarily produced by healthy persons (Table 5–1 on pages 34–35).[21]

A wide variety of urinary crystals are found. These are usually identified by their morphologic characteristics. However, physical, chemical, and staining properties may be of importance in specific identification. Abnormal crystals are most often found in urinary sediments with an acid or neutral pH. On the other hand, the normal crystals found in routine human sediment may be associated with urinary pH values that range from strongly acid to alkaline (Table 5–2). A discussion of crystals found in urinary sediments from both normal subjects and patients follows.

TABLE 5–2.—Normal Urinary Crystals

ACID URINE
Uric acid
Amorphous urates
Calcium oxalate
Hippuric acid
ALKALINE URINE
Amorphous phosphates
Triple phosphate
Calcium phosphate
Calcium carbonate
Ammonium urate

NORMAL CRYSTALS OF URINARY SEDIMENT

Uric Acid Crystals

Uric acid crystals are the most common of the crystalline forms encountered in urinary sediment. Although uric acid tends to crystallize more readily in very acidic urine, almost any acid urine allowed to stand at room temperature for a sufficient length of time will demonstrate uric acid crystal deposition. These crystals display

TABLE 5–1.—Urinary Crystals

CRYSTAL	COLOR	SHAPE	pH OF URINE	SOLUBLE IN	INSOLUBLE IN
		NORMAL CRYSTALS			
Uric acid	Yellow (most common), colorless, reddish brown	Rhombic, whetstone, spears, needles, barrels	Acid	NaOH, heat (slight)	HCl, CH_3COOH, alcohol
Amorphous urates	Yellowish red, pink (sediment)	Amorphous, granules	Acid, neutral	NaOH, heat	HCl, CH_3COOH
Calcium oxalate	Colorless	Octahedral, dumbbell, round	Acid, neutral, slightly alkaline	Dilute HCl, HNO_3, NaOH (slight), heat	CH_3COOH
Hippuric acid	Colorless, pale yellow	Needles, rhombic plates, six-sided prisms	Acid, neutral, slightly alkaline	NaOH, heat, ether, alcohol	CH_3COOH
Amorphous phosphate	Colorless, white (sediment)	Amorphous, granules	Neutral, alkaline	HCl, CH_3COOH	NaOH, heat
Triple phosphate	Colorless	Prisms (coffin lid), feathery	Neutral, alkaline	HCl, CH_3COOH	NaOH, heat
Calcium phosphate	Colorless	Flat irregular plates, wedge-shaped prisms, granules	Slightly acid, neutral, alkaline	HCl, CH_3COOH	NaOH, heat
Calcium carbonate	Colorless	Dumbbell, granules	Neutral, alkaline	HCl + $CO_2\uparrow$ CH_3COOH + $CO_2\uparrow$	NaOH, heat
Ammonium urate	Yellowish brown	Scorpion, thorn apple, spheres	Alkaline	NaOH + $NH_3\uparrow$ HCl, heat (slow)	

		ABNORMAL CRYSTALS			
Tyrosine	Colorless, yellow	Fine silky needles	Acid	NaOH, HCl, heat	CH_3COOH, alcohol, ether
Leucine	Yellowish brown	Spheroids with central striations	Acid	NaOH, hot CH_3COOH, heat	HCl, room temperature CH_3COOH, ether
Cystine	Colorless	Hexagonal plates	Acid	NaOH, HCl, NH_4OH	CH_3COOH, alcohol, ether, boiling H_2O
Cholesterol	Colorless	Flat plates with corners chipped out	Acid, neutral	$CHCl_3$, ether, hot alcohol	H_2O, dilute acids, dilute alkalis
Sulfa	Colorless, yellowish brown, greenish brown; colored complex formed by Lignin test	Amorphous, fan-shaped, shocks of wheat	Acid	Strong CH_3COOH, NaOH, acetone	Dilute CH_3COOH
Bilirubin	Bile-stained	Granules, needles	Acid	CH_3COOH, HCl, NaOH, $CHCl_3$, acetone, ether	
Starch	Colorless; purplish blue-black with iodine; does not stain with Sudan III	Irregularly round with dark striations to the center; asymmetric "Maltese cross" in polarized light; may be confused with leucine, fat bodies			

extreme pleomorphism in size and shape (Fig 5–1). Most frequently they appear yellow, but they may vary from reddish brown to colorless. Uric acid crystals are the great imposters of the urinary sediment, as they mimic the forms of many other crystals (Fig 5–2). They display birefringence when observed with polarized light (Fig 5–3). Shapes routinely encountered include whetstone, rhombic and six-sided plates, rosettes, stars, spears or clubs, needles, and barrels (Figs 5–4 and 5–5).

When heated, uric acid crystals are slightly soluble. They become readily soluble upon addition of an alkali such as sodium hydroxide. (Ammonium hydroxide is rarely employed as an alkali in this instance, because the reaction promotes the formation of ammonium urate crystals.) Uric acid crystals are insoluble in alcohol, acetic acid, and hydrochloric acid.

The quantity of dietary purines and the catabolism of nucleic acids are reflected by the uric acid content of urine. Uric acid crystals are considered pathologic only when they appear in a freshly voided specimen. In such instances their presence may indicate increased nucleoprotein metabolism, as is found in diseases such as gout or leukemia; impaired oxidation power, as encountered in respiratory-circulatory diseases; acute febrile conditions; or various forms of chronic renal disease. Uric acid crystals are of no clinical significance when found in urine that has cooled.

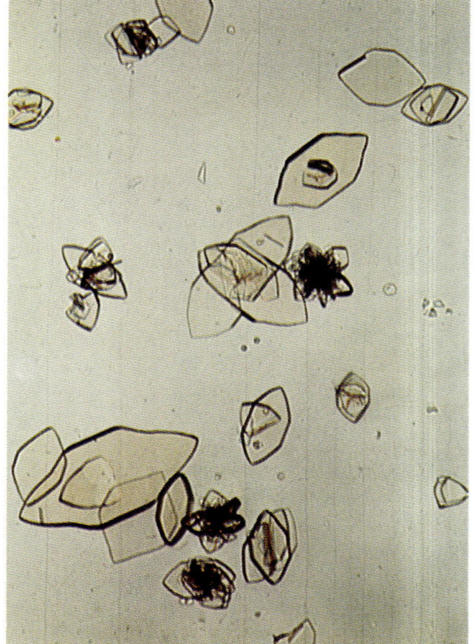

Fig 5–1. Uric acid crystals. Note variegated appearance (BF ×160).

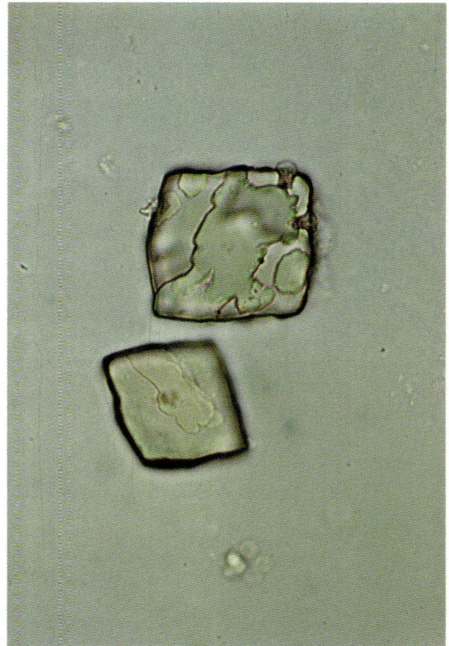

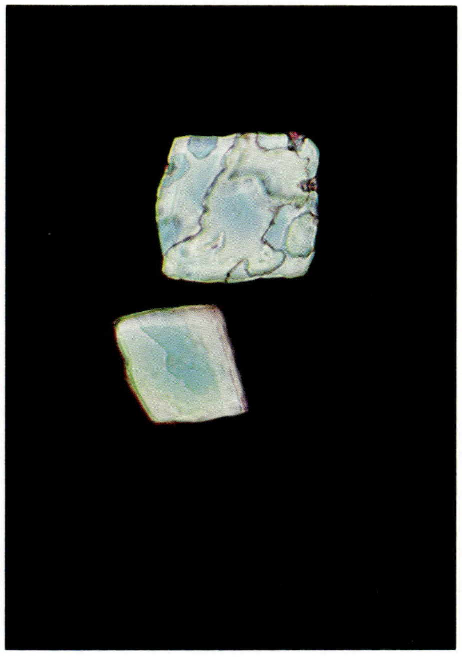

Fig 5–2 ***(left).*** High-power view of uric acid crystals assuming four-sided plate form (BF ×160).
Fig 5–3 ***(right).*** Same crystals as seen in Figure 5–2, but with polarized light. Urate crystals show birefringence (Pol ×160).

Amorphous Urates

Amorphous urates are salts of uric acid and are found in acid or neutral urine. These salts frequently precipitate in urine that has been refrigerated or has cooled to room temperature. These urates are pink, tan, or yellowish red and appear as amorphous or granular forms (Fig 5–6). They may be present in such large amounts that they obscure other formed elements in the sediment. In such instances they should be "cleared" before microscopic examination.

Clearing the sediment of amorphous urates is done by centrifuging an aliquot of urine (usually 10–12 ml), decanting, replacing the supernatant with an equal volume of a warm saline solution, and then mixing and centrifuging the specimen again. The sediment is then ready to be examined. The warm saline acts to dissolve and dilute the urates. Uric acid granules are also soluble when heated gently in the presence of an alkali such as sodium hydroxide. They are generally insoluble in acids, but may dissolve slightly to form uric acid. Observed most often in concentrated urine, amorphous urates usually have no clinical significance.

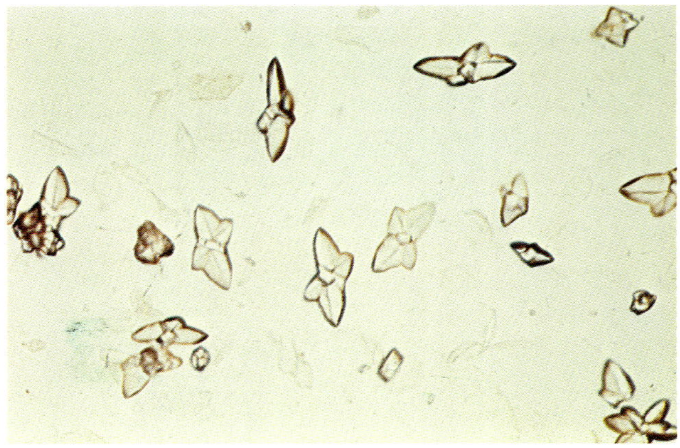

Fig 5–4. Star-shaped urate crystals (BF ×160).

Calcium Oxalate Crystals

Calcium oxalate crystals are usually found in acid urine but may also be formed in urine having a pH that is slightly alkaline or neutral. These crystals occur in two basic structural shapes, the octahedral and the dumbbell; other shapes are variants of these two forms (Figs 5–7 and 5–8).

Oxalate crystals are soluble in dilute hydrochloric acid and in 90% ethyl alcohol but are insoluble in acetic acid. The octahedral form of calcium oxalate crystals occurring in slightly alkaline urine may be easily mistaken for triple phosphate. These two crystals can be differentiated by their solubility properties. Triple phosphate is readily soluble in acetic acid, whereas calcium oxalate is not. The most significant identification problem of the calcium oxalate crystal occurs when it ap-

Fig 5–5. Spear-shaped uric acid crystals in urine sediment (BF ×160).

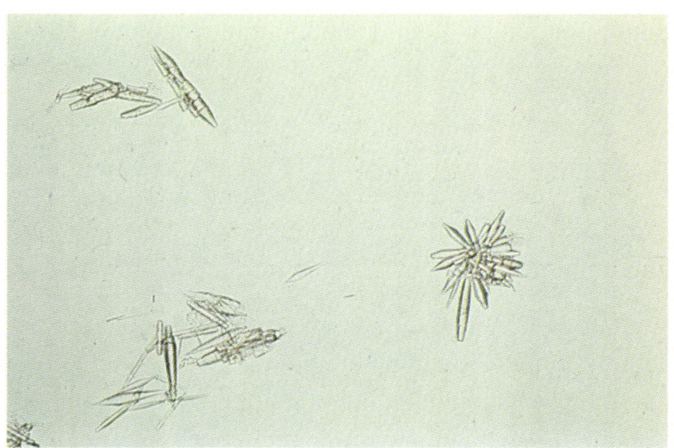

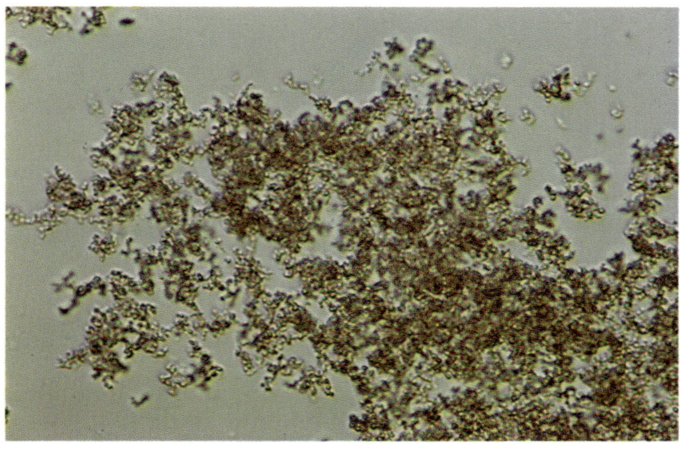

Fig 5–6. Amorphous urates, which appear as fine, brownish tan granules (BF ×200).

Fig 5–7 ***(left).*** Calcium oxalate crystals, which are commonly octahedral. Squamous cell is shown for size comparison (BF ×100).

Fig 5–8 ***(right).*** Variegated forms of calcium oxalate crystals, including dumbbell and ovoid or elliptic (BF ×160).

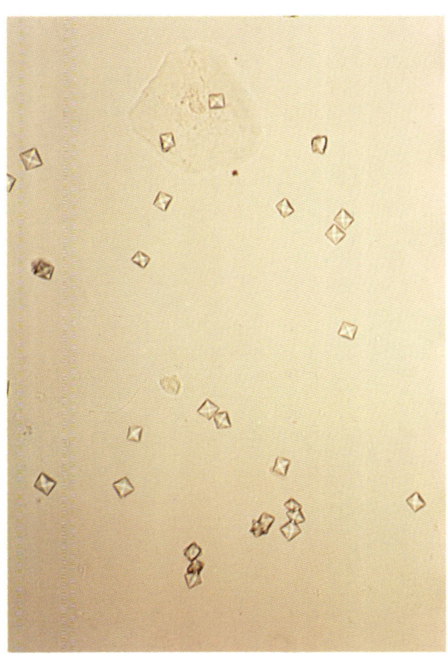

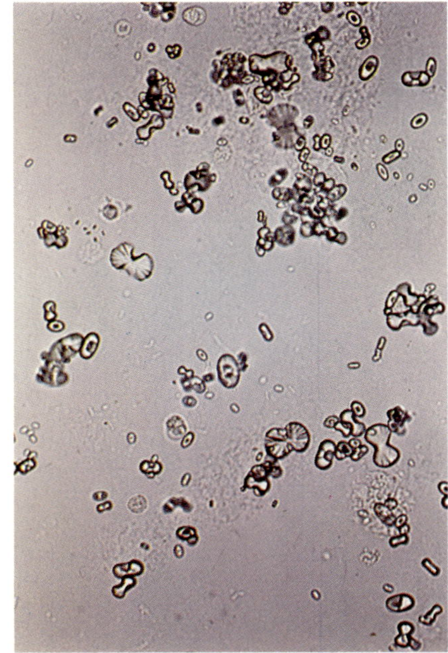

pears in a round or oval form and resembles red blood cells. Round oxalate crystals are biconcave, highly refractive, polarize light, and are insoluble in acetic acid. Red blood cells are lysed in acetic acid and do not polarize light.

All forms of calcium oxalate crystals may be found in normal urine, depending on the subject's diet. They tend to occur in increasing numbers when foods rich in oxalic acid (tomatoes, apples, asparagus, oranges, or carbonated beverages) are consumed in large quantities. These crystals have a high potential for forming renal calculi and may be seen in greater numbers in patients with pathologic conditions such as diabetes mellitus, heart-lung diseases, diseases of the nervous system, and organic diseases of the liver.

Hippuric Acid Crystals

Hippuric acid crystals are rarely found in urine. They may form when the urine is neutral or slightly alkaline but are most frequently found in acidic urine. Crystals of hippuric acid are colorless or pale yellow and occur as six-sided prisms, needles, or rhombic plates (Fig 5–9). They are soluble in sodium hydroxide, ether, alcohol, and hot water, and are insoluble in acetic acid.

Hippuric acid crystals are produced in the normal subject after the ingestion of fruits and vegetables that contain large quantities of benzoic acid. They are usually of no clinical significance. However, patients suffering from hepatic diseases and acute febrile conditions have been reported to have hippuric acid crystals in their urine.

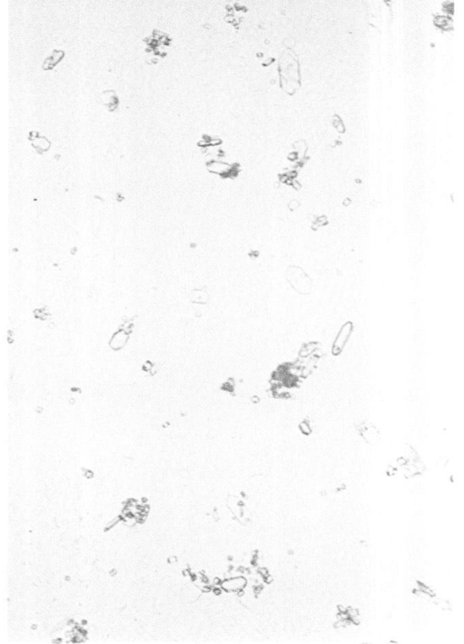

Fig 5–9. Hippuric acid crystals (BF ×160).

Amorphous Phosphates

Amorphous phosphates appear in neutral to alkaline urine as fine, colorless, or slightly brown granules (Fig 5–10). They tend to aggregate into groups or clumps, especially on refrigeration of the urine, and obscure any formed elements of the urinary sediment that might be present. In urine containing amorphous phosphates, white precipitate is observed on centrifugation. As in instances where amorphous urates are found, amorphous phosphate granules should also be cleared before microscopic examination of the sediment is performed.

Amorphous phosphate crystals are soluble in acetic acid, and one or two drops of this acid added to the sediment is sufficient to clear them. However, the urine sediment should be examined for the presence of red blood cells before the addition of acetic acid, since these cells will be lysed after the acid has been added. Amorphous phosphates are insoluble on heating. This fact helps to differentiate them from amorphous urates. These phosphates generally appear in the urine during the alkaline tide following a heavy meal and are of no clinical significance.

Triple Phosphate Crystals

Triple phosphate crystals, also known as ammonium magnesium phosphate, are often present in alkaline or neutral urine. They are colorless, usually have a prismatic form, and display birefringence in polarized light (Figs 5–11 and 5–12). The prisms have been described as looking like "coffin lids."

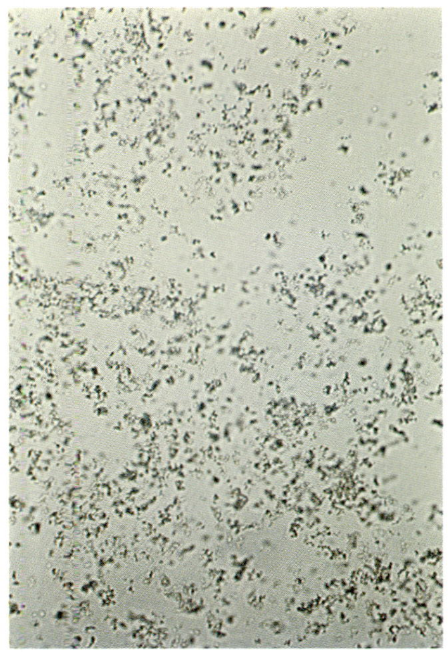

Fig 5–10. Amorphous phosphate crystals (BF ×160).

These crystals are soluble in acetic acid and may assume a feathery or leaflike appearance upon going into solution (Fig 5–13). Usually they have no clinical significance. However, the presence of triple phosphate crystals in the sediment of a fresh urine specimen may be due to the action of a urea-splitting microorganism, possibly secondary to urinary tract obstruction or stasis.

Calcium Phosphate Crystals

Calcium phosphate crystals, also known as dicalcium phosphate or stellate phosphate crystals, appear most often in alkaline urine but may also appear in neutral or slightly acid urine. They may have granular, amorphous, or crystalline forms (Fig 5–14). The most common form is a large, flat, and irregular crystal resembling a sheet of ice. These crystals may also appear as wedge-shaped prisms, either singly or in rosettes.

Fig 5–11 ***(left).*** Triple phosphate crystals in urine, resembling prisms or "coffin lids" (ICM ×160).
Fig 5–12 ***(right).*** Triple phosphate crystals in urine. This is the same field of view as shown in Figure 5–11. Note birefringence (Pol ×160).

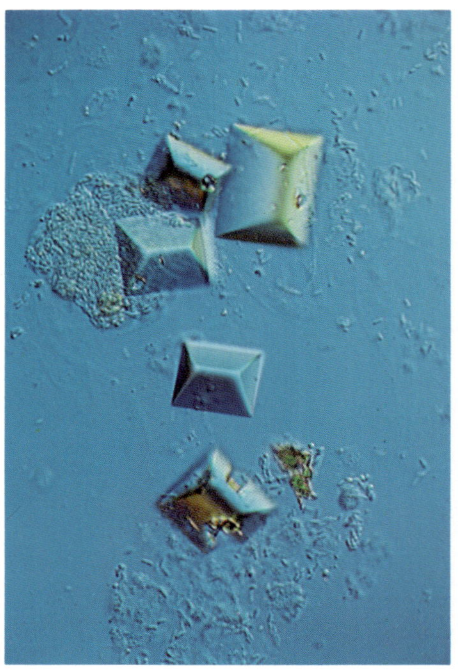

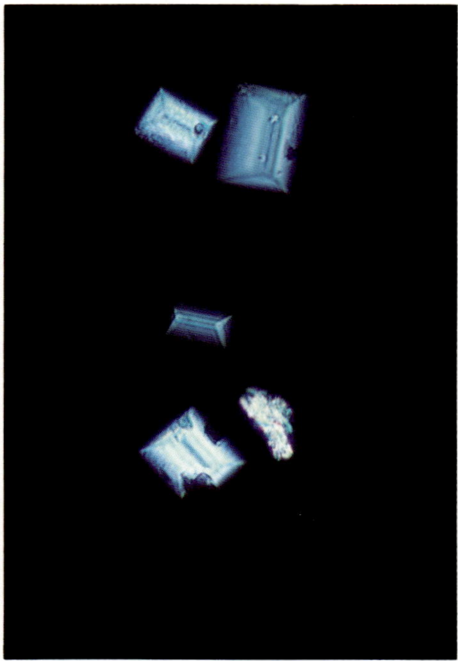

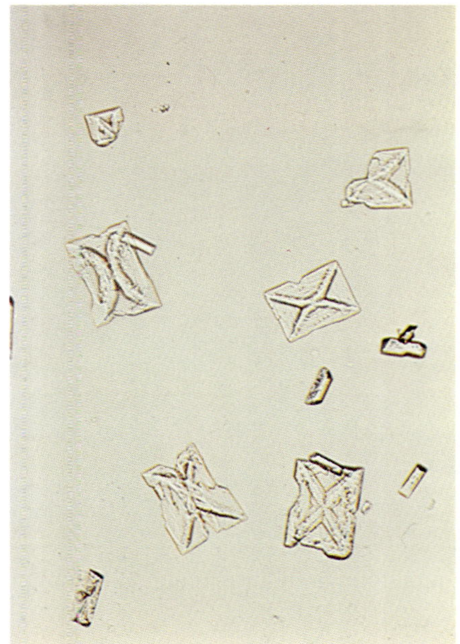

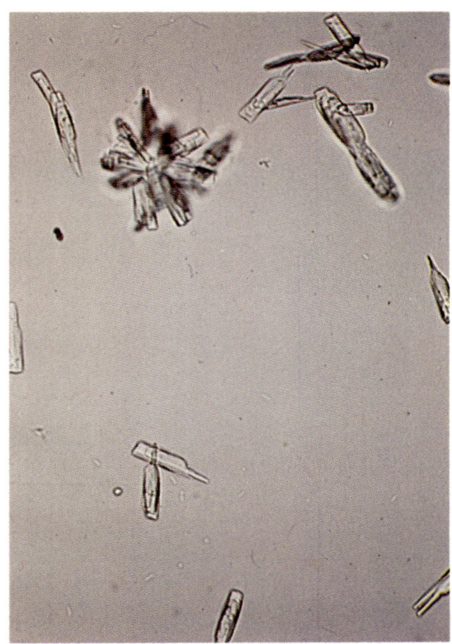

Fig 5–13 *(left).* Feathery form of triple phosphate crystals in urine (BF ×160).
Fig 5–14 *(right).* Calcium phosphate crystals, assuming variable forms, including rosette, plate, and pointed finger shown here (BF ×160).

When the urine is heated, the amorphous form of calcium phosphate crystals precipitates. This test should not be confused with the heat test for protein with protein precipitation. It can be distinguished from the protein test by acidifying the urine with acetic acid before performing the protein determination. In such instances, interference with the protein test by calcium phosphate crystals can be alleviated, since these crystals are soluble in acetic acid.

Calcium phosphate crystals usually have no clinical significance, although they are commonly observed in the urine of patients with cystitis associated with urine retention. These crystals have the potential for forming renal calculi and tend to irritate the urinary tract when formed within the body.

Calcium Carbonate Crystals

Calcium carbonate crystals are small and colorless and appear in alkaline urine as granules or as small dumbbells (Figs 5–15 and 5–16). The addition of acetic or hydrochloric acid to sediment containing calcium carbonate crystals causes their dissolution, with subsequent bubbling and the release of carbon dioxide.

Calcium carbonate crystals appear in urinary sediment after the ingestion of large quantities of vegetables and have no clinical significance.

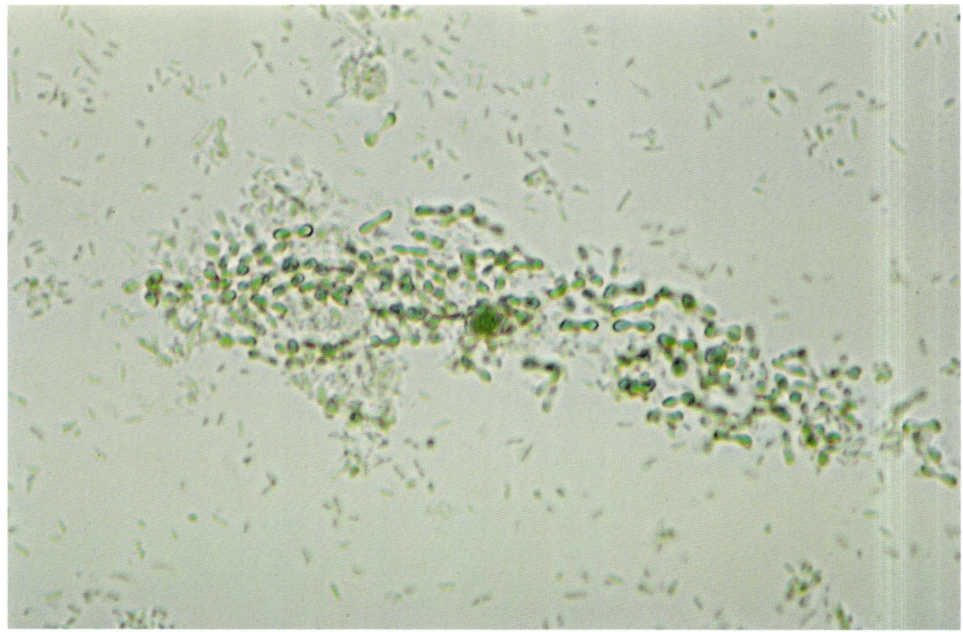

Fig 5–15. Calcium carbonate crystals, which invariably occur as small, colorless dumbbells. Bacteria are also present for comparison (BF ×250).

Fig 5–16. Calcium carbonate crystals in urine—polarized, birefringent, and thus distinguished from various microorganisms. This is the same field as shown in Figure 5–15 (Pol ×250).

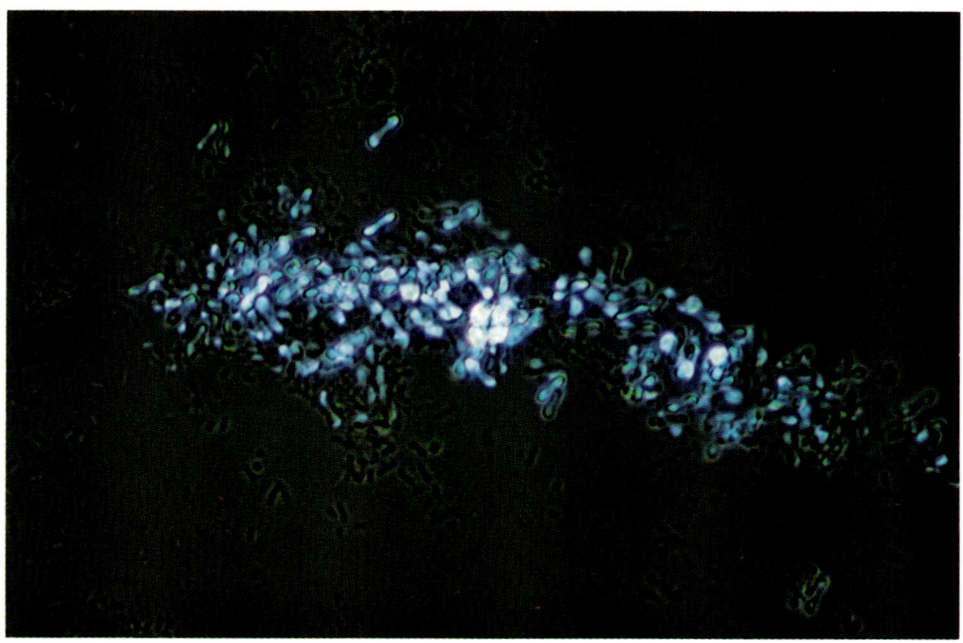

Ammonium Urates

Ammonium urates are the only urate crystals that occur in alkaline urine. They are yellowish brown and assume two basic forms—either spheroids or spheres with radiating spicules (Fig 5–17). The latter shape is frequently referred to as "thorn apple," and the crystal is said to resemble a scorpion. The two forms often appear together in urinary sediments.

Ammonium urate crystals are soluble in sodium hydroxide, and ammonia gas is evolved as they dissolve. When acetic or hydrochloric acid is added to urine containing these urate crystals, they dissolve slowly and are replaced by uric acid crystals. Ammonium urate crystals dissolve slowly when heated and recrystallize on cooling.

Ammonium urate crystals are considered to have no clinical significance but often form when there is ammonia formation in urine present in the bladder (ie, in bacterial cystitis).

ABNORMAL CRYSTALS OF URINARY SEDIMENT

The importance of recognizing normal crystals in the urine is due to the fact that without this knowledge a clear delineation of abnormal crystals uncommonly found in the sediment (but nevertheless of great importance) cannot be made. The crystals herein presented and described are those of the abnormal type that are found in acid urine predominantly. Most are infrequently seen.

Fig 5–17. Ammonium urate crystals, easily distinguished by their golden brown color and "thorn apple" shape (BF ×160).

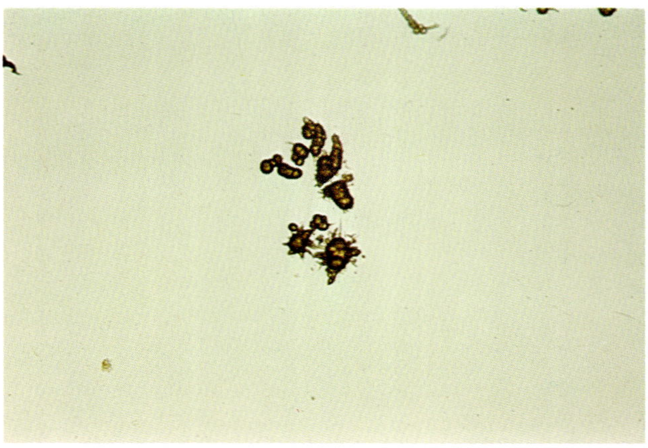

Tyrosine Crystals

Crystals of tyrosine are rarely observed in the urine and are present only when the urine is acid. They are colorless to yellowish brown, needle-shaped crystals and have a fine silky appearance (Fig 5–18). The needles may be single or arranged in sheaves or rosettes. Tyrosine crystals usually appear in urinary sediment together with leucine. They are soluble in hydrochloric acid, sodium hydroxide, and boiling water, and insoluble in alcohol, ether, and acetic acid.

Leucine and tyrosine are both products of protein metabolism and may appear in the urine of patients with tissue degeneration or necrosis (eg, acute liver disease due to hepatitis virus; certain hepatocellular poisons such as phosphorus, chloroform, or carbon tetrachloride; cirrhosis of the liver; obstructive jaundice; and severe cases of leukemia, typhoid fever, and smallpox).

Leucine Crystals

Leucine crystals are found in acidic urine in the form of spheroids with concentric striations (Fig 5–19). They are dense and highly refractile and appear as yellowish brown bodies, sometimes oily looking, which may cause them to be confused with free fat bodies. Leucine spheres are birefringent and polarize light, demonstrating a pseudo-"Maltese cross" appearance when polarized light is used (Fig 5–20). Leucine crystals are soluble in sodium hydroxide, hot acetic acid, and hot water, and insoluble in ether and in hydrochloric and acetic acids at room temperature.

Although rare, leucine crystals often appear in the urine in association with tyrosine and are manifestations of the same clinical conditions.

Fig 5–18. Tyrosine crystals (BF ×160).

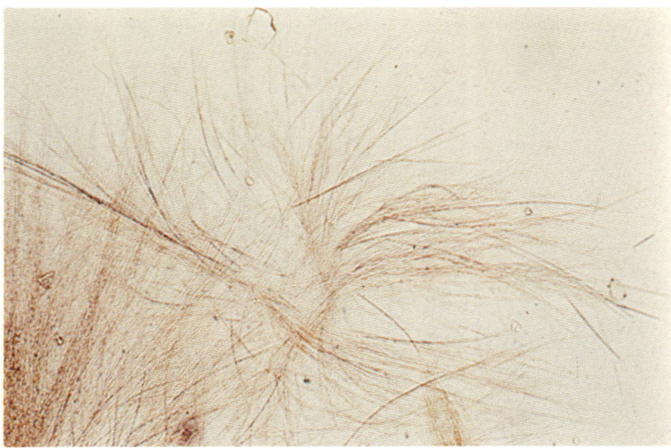

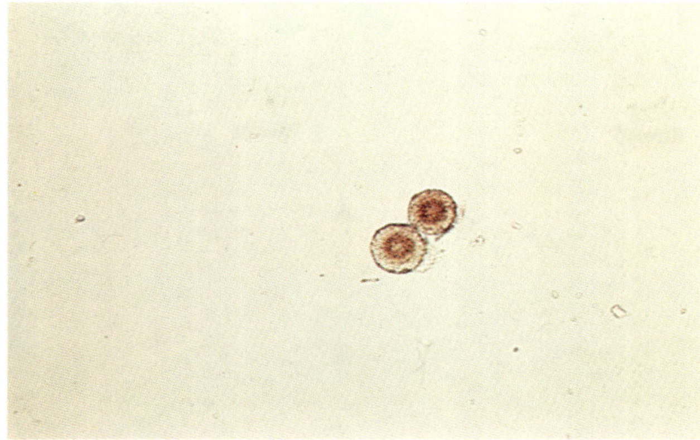

Fig 5–19. Leucine crystals, which are highly refractile and characterized by central concentric ring configuration with radiating spokes (BF ×160).

Cystine Crystals

Cystine, an amino acid, is rarely a constituent of urine. Cystine crystals are observed in urine with an acid pH and are seen as thin, colorless, hexagonal plates, usually with two sides longer or shorter than the other four; occasionally they may assume other configurations, however (Fig 5–21). Frequently the plates will overlie one another or fuse into a rosette. They are usually flat or platelike, and when dissolving, become wrinkled and somewhat globular. They are ordinarily colorless and display birefringence with polarized light. Cystine crystals are soluble in hydrochloric acid, sodium hydroxide, and ammonium hydroxide; and insoluble in acetic acid, ether, alcohol, and boiling water.

Fig 5–20. Leucine crystals in urine, demonstrating birefringence and pseudo-"Maltese-cross" appearance. These are the same crystals shown in Figure 5–19 (Pol ×160).

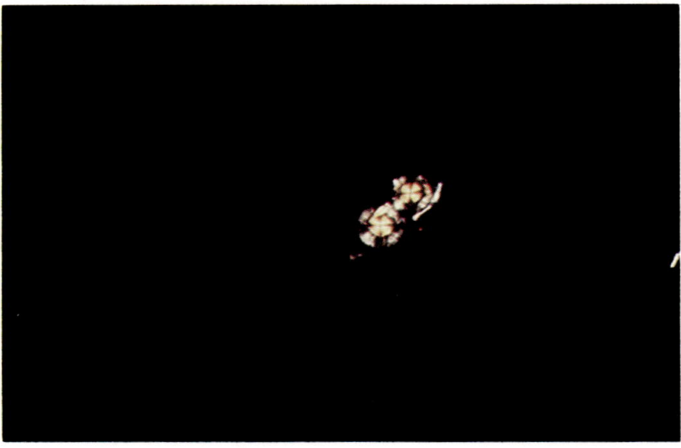

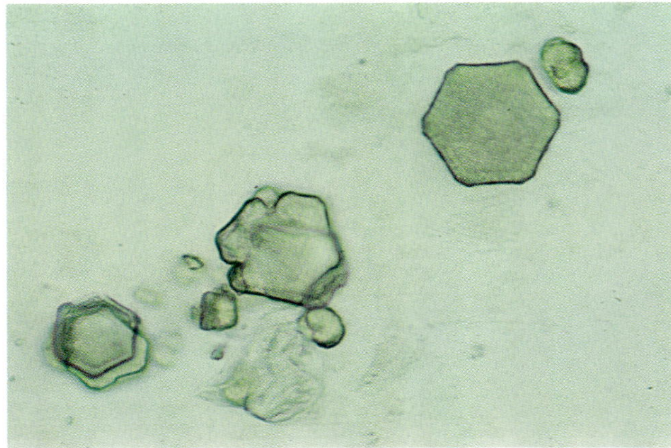

Fig 5–21. Cystine crystals in urine. Note characteristic hexagonal, platelike, colorless features (BF ×160).

Cystine crystals are most often observed in the urine of patients suffering from a variety of hereditary-familial metabolic disorders involving the renal transport of various amino acids such as cystine, lysine, arginine, and ornithine.

Cholesterol Crystals

Cholesterol crystals are found in acid or neutral urine. They appear as regular or irregular transparent plates. They may occur singly or in large numbers and are birefringent in polarized light. Usually one or more of the corners are cut off or notched, justifying their description as "stairstep crystals" (Figs 5–22 and 5–23). Cholesterol crystals may be found floating on top of the centrifuged urine specimen (supernatant) as well as in the sediment. The crystals are soluble in chloroform, ether, and boiling alcohol, and are insoluble in dilute acids and alkalis.

Cholesterol crystals are uncommonly seen in urine and are always considered pathologic. They can be found in various renal diseases, the nephrotic syndrome, or in other conditions in which there is formation or deposition of lipids in the kidney.

Bilirubin Crystals

Bilirubin crystals appear in acidic urine as pigmented yellowish brown granules or clusters of needles (Figs 5–24 and 5–25). They are soluble in acetic and hydrochloric acids, sodium hydroxide, acetone, chloroform, and ether.

Bilirubin crystals are considered pathologic and may be found in the urine of patients suffering from a wide variety of hepatobiliary and hematopoietic diseases in which clinical jaundice is often a prominent symptom.

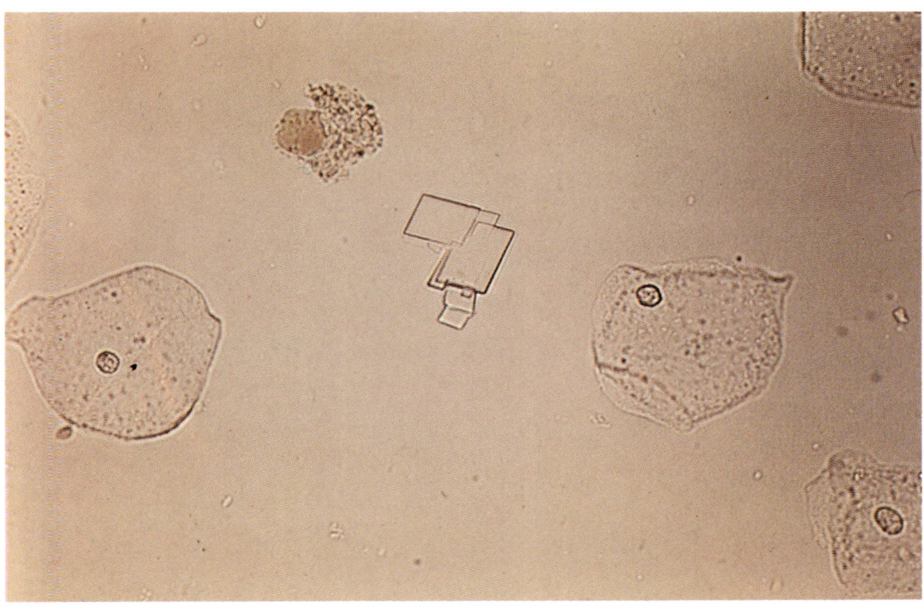

Fig 5–22. Cholesterol crystals. These irregular transparent plates are among the easiest crystals to recognize, as they often have a notched corner. Two squamous epithelial cells are shown at either side of the crystals (BF ×160).

Fig 5–23. Cholesterol crystals, showing birefringence. Note variegated appearance but consistency of plate form (Pol ×160).

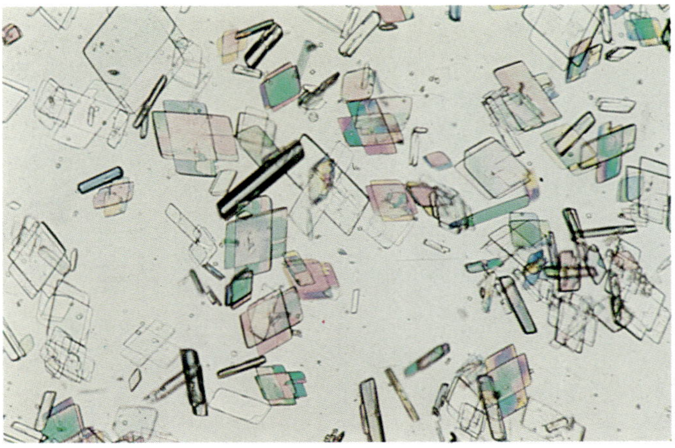

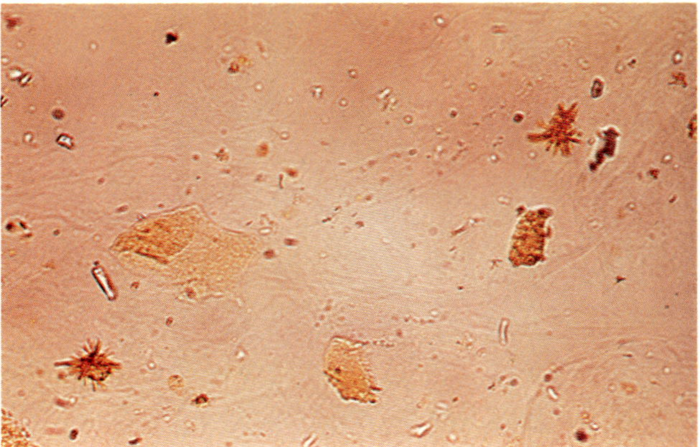

Fig 5–24. Bilirubin crystals, which are single or grouped in clusters of brown spicules, often projecting from central nidus. Note two squamous epithelial cells towards the center (BF ×160).

Hemosiderin

Granules of hemosiderin occur in the urine infrequently. They are fine, reddish brown granules (Fig 5–26), but they may be difficult to distinguish from certain other granules such as amorphous urates or phosphates. Hemosiderin granules are not birefringent in polarized light and can easily be stained for the presence of iron, using Turnbull's blue or Prussian blue techniques wherein the iron exhibits a dark blue color (Fig 5–27).

Fig 5–25. Bilirubin granules and clusters in urine. Note brown pigmentation of these crystals (BF ×160).

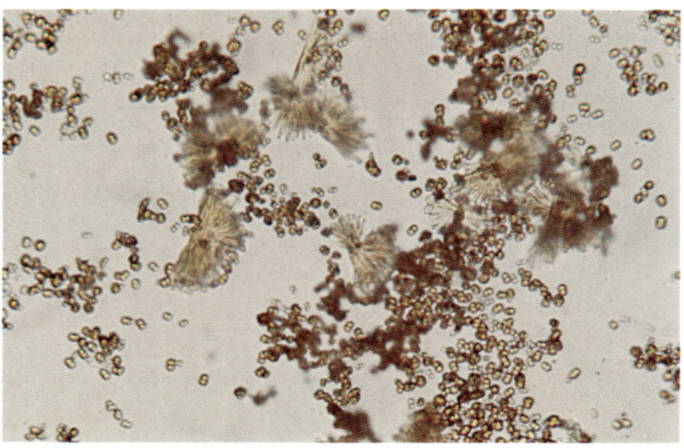

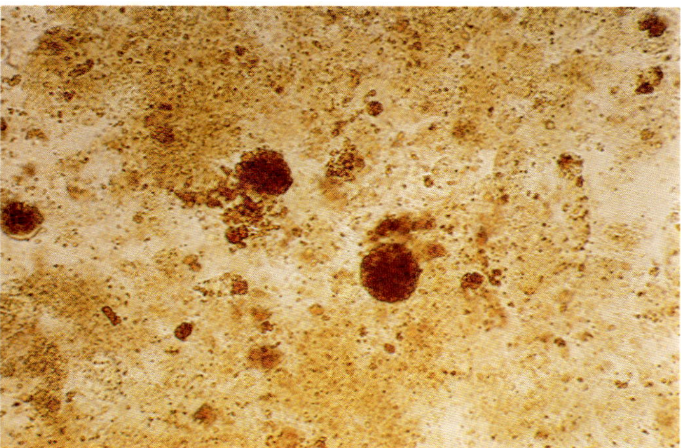

Fig 5–26. Reddish brown hemosiderin granules of various sizes. Some are aggregated into larger globules, but most are single and somewhat spheric. Polarization would show absence of birefringent properties, thus distinguishing these granules from amorphous urates or phosphates (BF ×100).

Hemosiderin is present in the urine in conditions causing severe hemolysis such as hemolytic anemia, transfusion reactions, and certain acute bacterial infections such as gas gangrene (caused by the organism *Clostridium perfringens*). In such cases the urine is discolored, cloudy, assumes a reddish tint, and contains measurable protein. The patient is usually severely ill or moribund.

Fig 5–27. Hemosiderin granules in microscopic field similar to that of Figure 5–26. The urine has been stained with Prussian blue dye, producing a blue color in the iron pigment in the hemoglobin molecule, a part of hemosiderin (BF ×100).

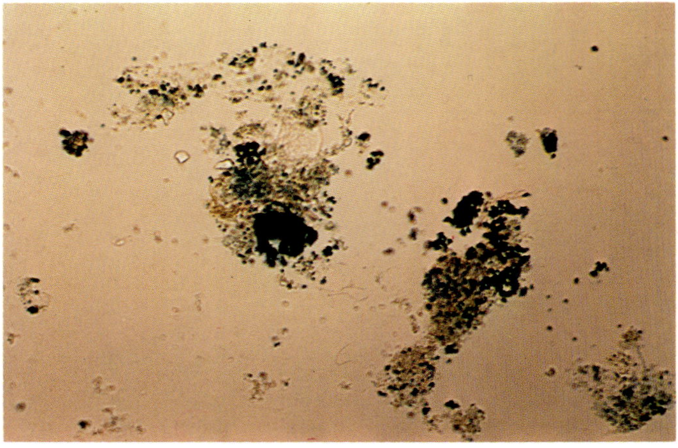

Sulfonamide Crystals

Sulfonamide crystals form primarily in acid urine. The shape and color of these crystals may be extremely variable, depending on the particular sulfonamide being administered to the patient. Sulfa crystals vary from colorless to greenish brown or yellowish brown to brown. The shape of these crystals ranges from amorphous granules to well formed plates, whetstones, and hexagons, which are morphologically indistinguishable from the crystals of uric acid. However, the most common forms encountered include rosettes, fan shapes, and those resembling shocks of wheat (Figs 5–28 through 5–30). Sulfonamide crystals are soluble in acetone, strong acids, and strong alkalis such as acetic acid or sodium hydroxide. These crystals are insoluble in dilute acetic acid. A procedure to confirm the presence of a sulfonamide in urine is the *Lignin test*. One drop of urine is placed on newspaper, after which one drop of 10% hydrochloric acid is added. The area is observed for a yellowish orange color, which is a positive confirmation of the presence of sulfonamides in the urine. Color development may take as long as fifteen minutes.

Sulfonamide crystals have pathologic significance, since they tend to form renal calculi that may damage renal tubules, especially when hydration of the patient is less than optimal.

Fig 5–28 ***(left).*** Sulfa crystals in urine, resembling a shock of wheat (BF ×160).
Fig 5–29 ***(right).*** Sulfa crystals in urine. Here they are needlelike, have a high refractive index, and often radiate from central focus (BF ×250).

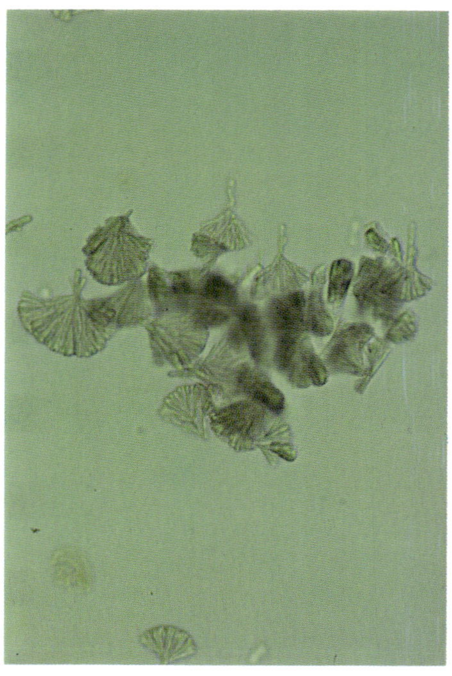

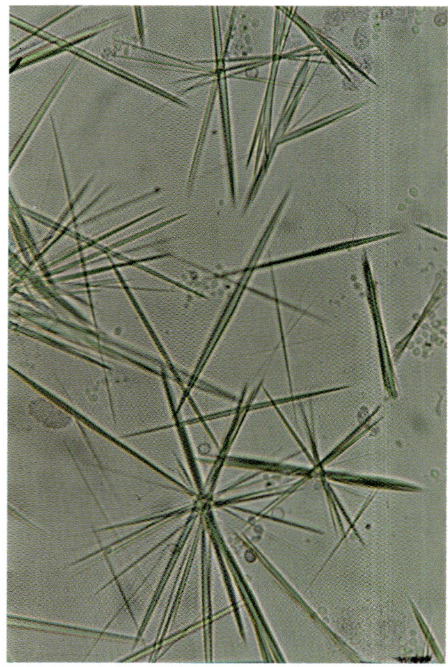

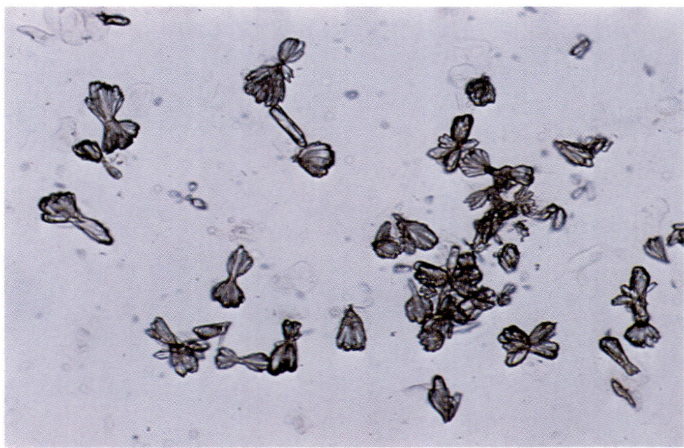

Fig 5–30. Another form of sulfa crystals (sulfisoxazole or Gantrisin) in urine (BF ×40).

Other Crystals Found in Urine

Many other crystals may be present in human urine, and no attempt is made in this text to cover them all. Often their presence is related to the administration of therapeutic or diagnostic compounds such as injection dyes used in intravenous pyelography (IVP). A few are illustrated in this chapter (Figs 5–31 and 5–32).

Fig 5–31. Intravenous pyelogram dye crystals in urine, which are thick, colorless, and birefringent when polarized. The IVP dye contains radiopaque iodine (BF ×160).

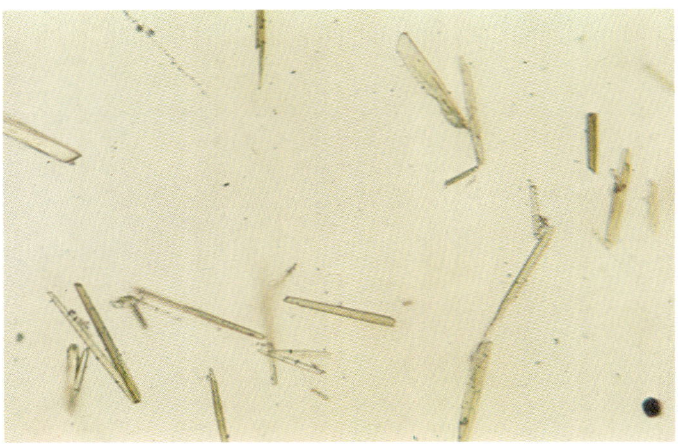

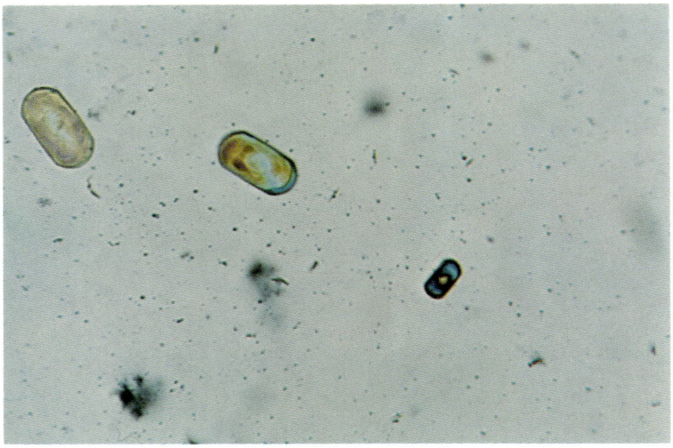

Fig 5–32. Acetaminophen (Tylenol) crystals in urine, resembling minute capsules. They show birefringence, have a high refractive index, and are uniformly shaped but vary in size (Pol ×160).

6. URINARY CASTS

Urinary casts may be defined as microscopic, cylindrically shaped formed elements of the urinary sediment that have been molded in the lumen of the renal tubule (usually the distal or collecting tubule). Casts are composed primarily of plasma proteins of the glomerular filtrate and a special mucoprotein (Tamm-Horsfall mucoprotein) secreted into the urine by tubular epithelial cells of the ascending portion of the loop of Henle.[40-42, 46, 60] Once formed, they pass from the collecting duct into the renal pelvis and then by way of the urinary stream through the ureter into the bladder, and exit from the body via the urethra. Casts are perhaps the most prognostically significant of all elements found in the urinary sediment. Often they mirror diseases of the kidneys and accurately reflect the course and prognosis of a specific renal disease. *Cylindruria* is another name for the presence of casts in the urine.

Casts in the urine of an otherwise healthy person are not necessarily prognosticators of disease. Recent studies have shown that hyaline and granular casts may be present in normal urine in relatively large numbers.[23] Most often this cast-forming response of the kidneys is directly related to an antecedent physical stress such as playing a game of football or running a mile, or to an emotional stress. In such instances hyaline and granular casts are usually found in the sediment in varying numbers (from just a few per low-power field to as many as 30–50). In the normal subject, therefore, the presence or absence of hyaline and granular casts must be carefully assessed. A thorough clinical history may not always indicate whether or not the subject had undergone physical or emotional stress before the urinalysis specimen was obtained.

Hyaline or granular casts in healthy persons are usually not accompanied by a significant degree of proteinuria (ie, greater than 1+, using dipstick methodology).[20] In our studies, up to 3+ protein (130 mg/ml) was present in the urine of a few subjects after stress.[23] However, this degree of proteinuria, and for that matter any dipstick-measurable proteinuria, ordinarily disappears within 24 hours after the stressful event. The amount of proteinuria in healthy subjects after stress is generally related to their physical condition. Those in excellent physical "shape" excrete little or no protein; those in poor physical condition generally have the highest concentration of urinary protein after stress. To summarize, persistent proteinuria when accompanied by cylindruria is usually of pathologic significance. On the other hand, proteinuria related to a stressful situation and accompanied by cast formation will ordinarily disappear within 24 hours, when the urine shows a complete chemical reversion to normal.

The matrix of all casts is protein.[42] A specific mucoprotein, Tamm-Horsfall protein, and numerous other immunoproteins—for instance, many of the immunoglobulins, especially IgG and IgM—have been found to be components of urinary casts.[60] However, except for Tamm-Horsfall protein, no single specific immunoprotein in a cast has been associated exclusively with a specific disease entity.

Casts are classified on the basis of their microscopic appearance and whether or not they contain any cellular constituents.[21] A simple classification for urinary casts is shown in Table 6–1. Casts without cells may be classified as hyaline, granular, waxy, fatty, and pigmented. Casts with cells are identified by the type of cell included in their matrices. These cells originate either in the bloodstream (white blood cells or red blood cells) or in the kidney (renal tubular epithelial cells). In addition, a cast recognized some years ago, but the clinical importance of which had not been clearly established until recently, contains bacteria within its matrix and has been named the *bacterial cast*.[37] Finally, other elements that appear in the urine and simulate the appearance of urinary casts, such as crystals, have been named *pseudocasts*.[21, 63]

Casts change and their appearance alters as they pass through the nephron and the lower urinary tract. Direct observation of their modes of formation in situ in the kidney, as well as their varying characteristics in the urine, has led to the conclusion that many cellular casts during transit evolve into granular casts (Fig 6–1).[20] This is due to the fact that the cells in the cast matrix break down and lyse. With the dissolution of the cell, the nuclear and cytoplasmic components, without a supporting cell membrane or nuclear membrane, appear granular in the cast matrix. Therefore, the appearance of a cast at any one specific point in time may not truly reflect its origin or prior morphologic characteristics. This is especially true in patients with severe intrinsic renal disease in whom the renal transit time is significantly lengthened. In addition to cellular breakdown affecting the morphology of casts, it is thought that the protein matrix of the cast also changes. This may be due to the fact that certain protein components assume different morphologic characteristics under changing conditions of pH, osmotic pressure, and ionic charge.

Casts assume wide varieties of form within the urine. They may be elongate, tortuous, broad, thick, smooth, or wrinkled.[21, 51] Their morphologic shape depends very much on the environment in which they are made, as well as the length of transit time through the kidney and the physical characteristics of the urine. Each morphologic type of cast will be considered in detail on the following pages.

ACELLULAR CASTS

Hyaline Casts

These casts are frequently present in the urine of both healthy persons and patients with intrinsic renal disease.[21] Hyaline casts have also been found in the urine of patients receiving certain therapeutic and chemical agents that may not be directly related to renal disease but nevertheless affect the kidney. Examples of such drugs are diuretics and cation exchange resins.[17, 26]

Under normal conditions, hyaline casts are ordinarily present in relatively small numbers, but they may be increased greatly in the sediment within the first 24

TABLE 6–1.—Urinary Casts

TYPE	FEATURES
Acellular Casts	
Hyaline	Smooth or finely wrinkled surface, transparent, low index of refraction (hard to see), may be tortuous or coiled; basic matrix of all casts
Granular	Fine or coarse granules on surface, higher refractive index (easy to see); some originate from preexisting cellular casts; tortuosity rare
Waxy	Thick, opaque, high refractive index (easy to see), "broken-off" ends, notched parallel margins
Fatty	Yellowish tan fat globules of high refractive index on cast surface; polarization shows anisotropism
Pigment	Hyaline cast with adsorbed urine pigments, such as bile or hemoglobin, yellow to brown color, smooth or granular surface
Cellular Casts	
White blood cell	PMNs on surface of hyaline matrix, multilobed nuclei, granular cytoplasm
Red blood cell	RBCs on surface; hyaline matrix; cells may show disruption and hemoglobin pigmentation
Epithelial	Renal epithelial cells on hyaline matrix; single large nucleus per cell; cells may line up in rows
Bacterial	Cast surface covered with bacterial forms with or without PMNs; stains, phase- or interference-contrast microscopy show organisms
Mixed Casts	Combinations of above
Pseudocasts	Not a true cast, but closely packed crystals, cells, and mucus that resemble a cast

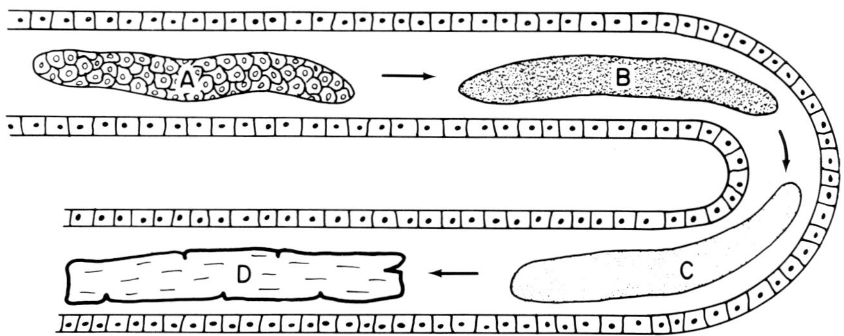

Fig 6–1. *(A)* Cellular cast, *(B)* granular cast, *(C)* finely granular cast, *(D)* waxy cast. (From Haber.[20] Used by permission.)

hours after severe mental or physical stress.[23] This type of cast presents as the classic prototype of all urinary casts, namely, as a transparent, cigar-shaped, cylindric gel of protein with smooth or finely wrinkled surfaces. It is beyond the scope of this text to enter into a prolonged discussion as to why and how hyaline casts form, and much of this information is unknown at present in any case; suffice it to say that hyaline casts are for the most part composed of proteinaceous fibrillar components, which have been identified by immunofluorescent techniques as Tamm-Horsfall proteins.[50]

Hyaline casts have a low refractive index and are colorless and transparent (Fig 6–2). They are difficult to see with an ordinary bright-field light microscope unless the contrast created by the microscopist is sufficient. Therefore, an inexperienced observer will often miss hyaline casts even when they are present if precautions are not taken or if special microscopic techniques are not used. It has been advocated that for the examination of urine sediment, specialized microscopic techniques such as phase-contrast or interference-contrast microscopy (Figs 6–3 and 6–4), or basic dyes for staining the sediment such as those included in the Sternheimer-Malbin stain (methyl violet and safranine) should be used routinely to avoid misdiagnosis.[11, 12, 18, 57] Once appropriate contrast is obtained, or the casts are visualized by one of the other enhancement techniques that capitalize on staining characteristics or differences in refractive index of the cast from the surrounding urine, hyaline casts appear as transparent, smooth, cylindrically-shaped elements of greatly varying size and configuration (Figs 6–5 and 6–6). In disease states, the casts may be "broad" (as compared with length), whereas under healthy conditions, hyaline casts are usually observed as elongate cylinders with curved ends. Past nomenclature has used the term *cylindroid* for a cast with a tapered end (see Fig 6–2).[21] This term

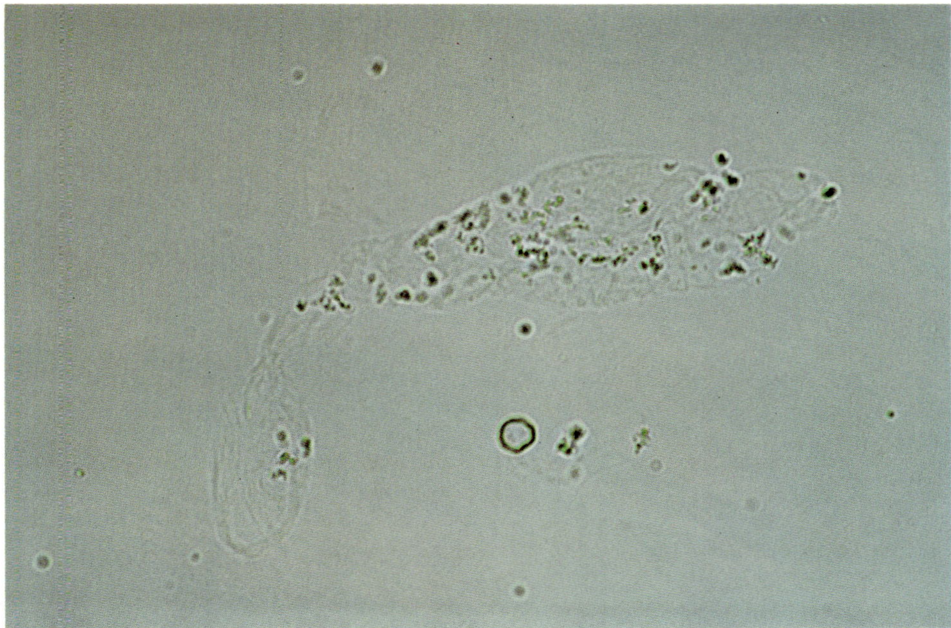

Fig 6–2. Hyaline cast. Though difficult to see due to its low refractive index, this one is granular, which makes visualization easier. Note that one end is "strung out." This form has been called "cylindroid" (BF ×200).

Fig 6–3. Hyaline cast, easily seen with phase-contrast microscopy. There are several mucus strands in the background. Fine granules are present on the cast surface (PH ×160).

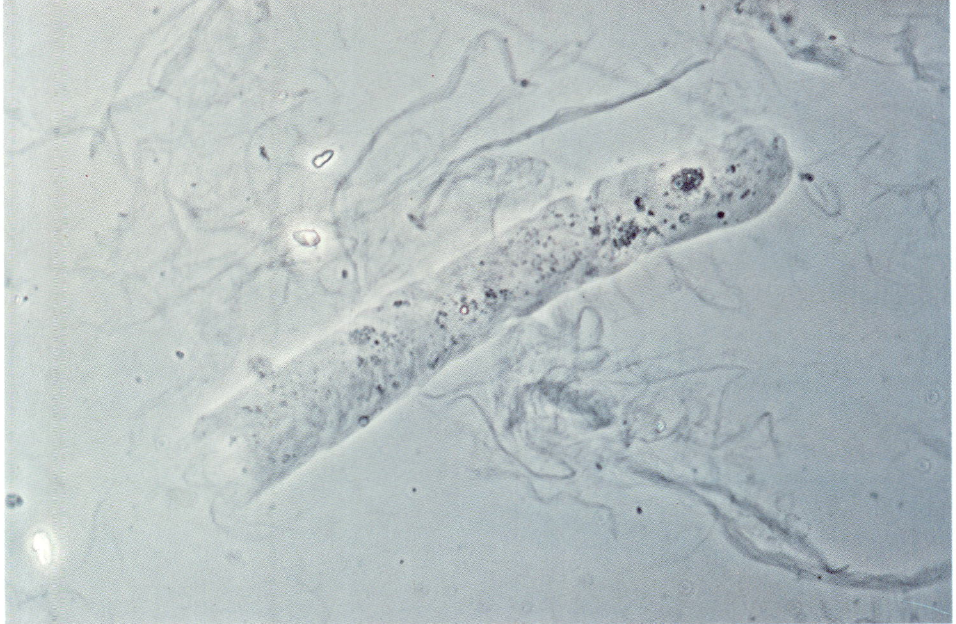

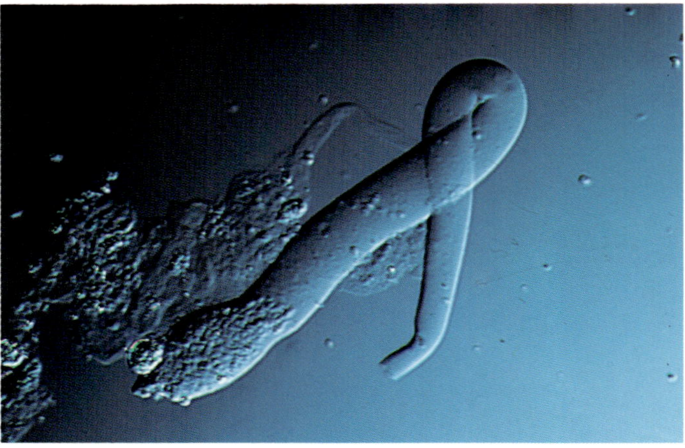

Fig 6–4. Hyaline cast. Note its tortuosity and granularity at one end (ICM ×200).

has no clinical significance, and hyaline casts in both disease and health often are seen as having long tapered ends.

In many hyaline casts various types of inclusions may be present within or on the matrix (Fig 6–7). These inclusions usually occur in the form of tiny granules, but may also be cellular parts such as nuclei or cell walls, blood cells, or fat droplets. One or two cells included in any given hyaline cast should not change the nomenclature assigned to the cast, ie, it is still a hyaline cast. In disease states, the type of cellular inclusion present in any given hyaline cast may provide some insight into the specific kind of renal disease the patient may have or into whether or not the patient does in fact have any intrinsic abnormality of the kidneys. For the most part, however, granules, and not cells, are most often observed in both normal and abnormal conditions. Granules may be coarse but are usually of the "fine"

Fig 6–5. Tortuous hyaline cast with some epithelial cells on the surface (BF ×250).

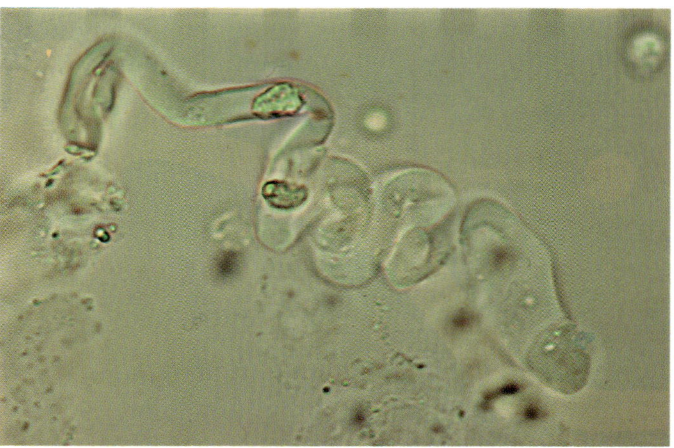

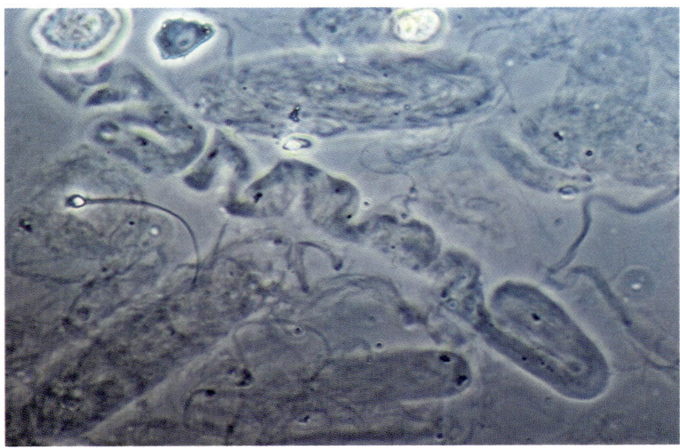

Fig 6–6. Hyaline casts in urine. Spermatozoa are also present (background). Diagonal cast is tortuous, whereas others are cigar-shaped and somewhat fibrillar (PH ×200).

type. The question as to the origin of the granules is presently unsolved, but it is apparent that granules in either a hyaline or a granular cast are not always associated with the breakdown of preexisting cells.

Electron microscopic study of hyaline casts has been most informative. Chapter 7 in this text has been devoted to the scanning electron microscopic (SEM) appearance of urinary casts, and the reader should consult it for further explanation. Suffice it to say at this time that the fibrillar protein meshwork of the hyaline cast is intricate and complex, and the specific environmental conditions in the nephron necessary for protein in the tubular lumen to coalesce and form fine filaments that comprise the cast are multifactorial. These conditions, at least in part, have to do with an appropriate electronic charge, pH, and ionic concentration of the urine.

When hyaline casts are present in a patient with intrinsic urinary tract disease, their morphologic complexity and numbers are usually increased above that which would be expected. Normally, a very small number (one or two per low-power field) of hyaline casts is present in the urinary sediment (except in stress). In disease this number may increase to as many as 30–50 per low-power field. When large numbers of hyaline casts are seen, therefore, the attending physician's attention should be called to the fact. As aforementioned, their increased production may be due to severe physical or emotional stress in the patient within the previous 24-hour period and is not necessarily due to an intrinsic renal abnormality.[23] *Athletic pseudonephritis,* a term coined to illustrate the clinical situation of cylindruria without accompanying intrinsic renal disease, has been appreciated in recent years because of current interest in jogging and other forms of strenuous physical activity that lead to abnormal urinary sediment findings.[7, 49] Often it may be difficult to distinguish normal from abnormal findings in such cases, and additional studies of renal function may be necessary.

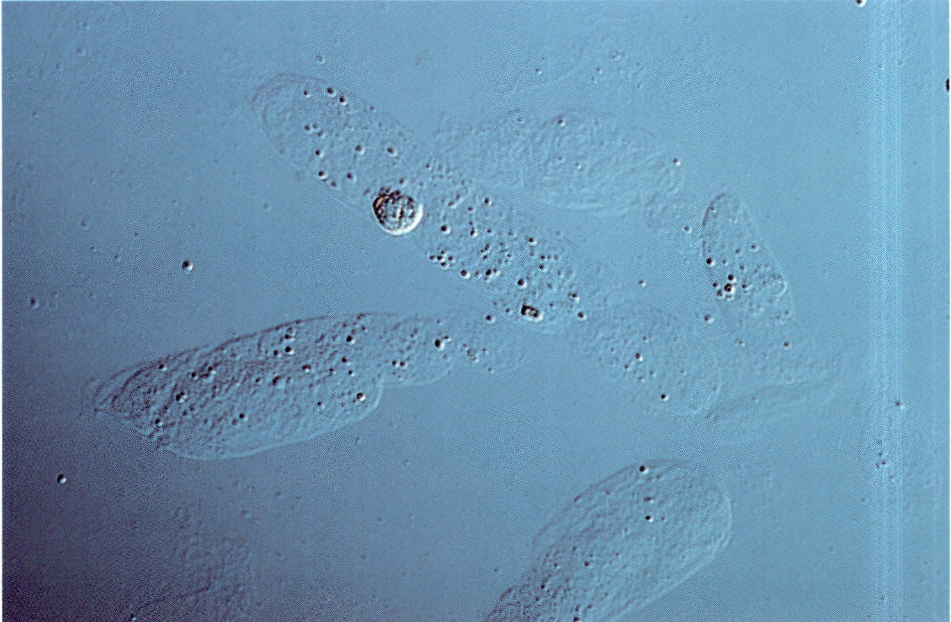

Fig 6–7. Hyaline casts with fine surface granules and delicate fibrils. One cast (center) contains cellular inclusion, probably a PMN. Note ease of visualization due to special microscopic technique (ICM ×160).

Granular Casts

Granular casts have morphologic characteristics very similar to those of hyaline casts. They are also present in the urine in both abnormal and normal states. Granular casts may be seen in large numbers after severe physical exercise on the part of healthy persons; on the other hand, they are frequently associated with nearly all forms of intrinsic renal disease. The origin of granular casts under normal conditions is unknown. However, since cellular casts are not part of the normal urinary sediment, it may be assumed that when granular casts appear in normal urinary sediment, they do not originate from the breakdown of preexistent cellular casts.

Cylindroid forms of granular casts occur relatively frequently. Again, as in the case of hyaline casts, they have no particular clinical significance. Granular casts, because of their inherent granularity, have a slightly higher refractive index than do hyaline casts; thus, they are much easier to see. Granules may be present throughout the entire cast matrix, confined to one area, or loosely scattered. The granules are often small and difficult to distinguish from one another, in which case the cast is called a *finely granular cast*, and the granules are considered *fine*. On the other hand, granules may be large, easily distinguished from one another, and are then called *coarse* granules (Figs 6–8 through 6–11). Distinguishing the fineness or coarseness of granules in any given cast has little clinical significance, however.

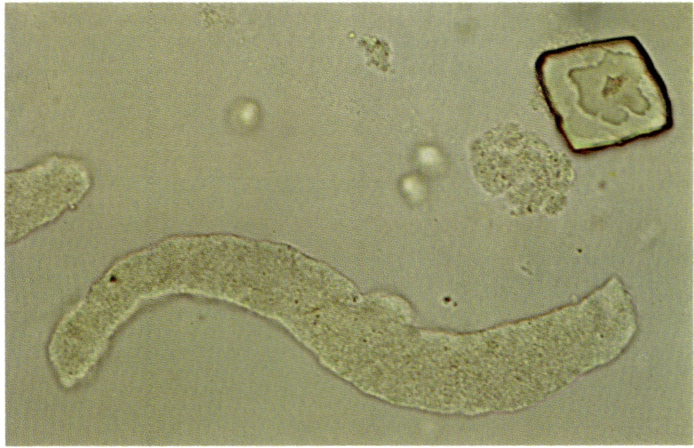

Fig 6–8. Finely granular cast in urine. Also, note uric acid crystal (BF ×160).

In the patient with intrinsic renal disease, it can be demonstrated that as cellular casts evolve during their transit through the nephron and the lower urinary tract, the constituent cells often break down and their nuclear and cytoplasmic constituents are observed as granules within the cast matrix (Fig 6–12). Evidence for this is striking and consists of finding nuclei or portions of nuclei and cell membranes still present in a matrix that is otherwise composed predominantly of granules. It has also been observed that as a granular cast evolves in the nephron, its morphology takes on a waxy appearance (Fig 6–13). It has a considerably higher refractive index than either granular or hyaline casts and has lost all or most of any preexistent cellular characteristics.

Fig 6–9. Broad, coarsely granular cast in urine. No vestiges of prior cellular origin (ie, cell cytoplasmic or nuclear components) are seen (Sternheimer-Malbin stain ×200).

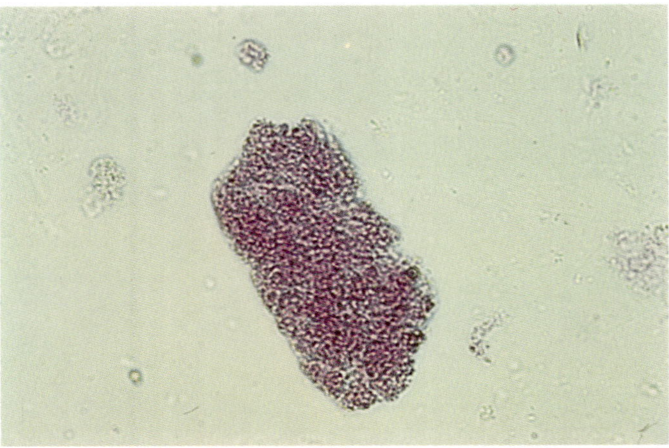

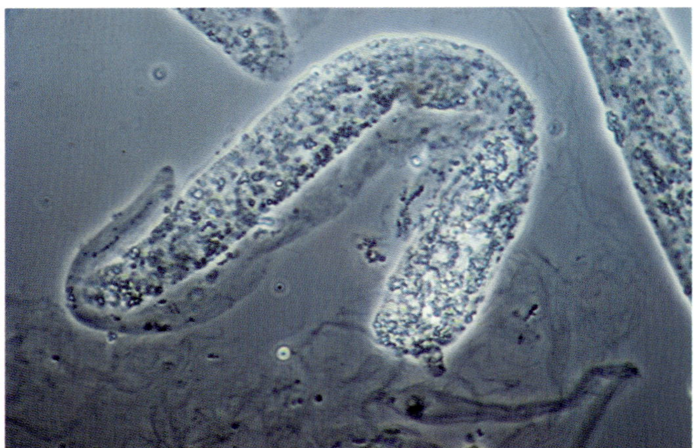

Fig 6–10. Granular casts with numerous mucus threads in the background (PH ×200).

A cast ordinarily misidentified as granular in type, the *bacterial cast*, has recently been shown to be composed of bacteria and not nonspecific granular material.[37] This differentiation is important, as the presence of bacterial casts in the urine is pathognomonic of pyelonephritis or intrinsic renal infection. To distinguish the granules from actual bacterial forms, staining of the sediment or special microscopic techniques (interference- or phase-contrast microscopy) enable the observer to recognize microorganisms specifically as integral components of the cast. Bacterial casts will be discussed at length later in a separate section of this chapter.

Fig 6–11. Coarse granular cast, easily seen with interference-contrast microscopy (ICM ×160).

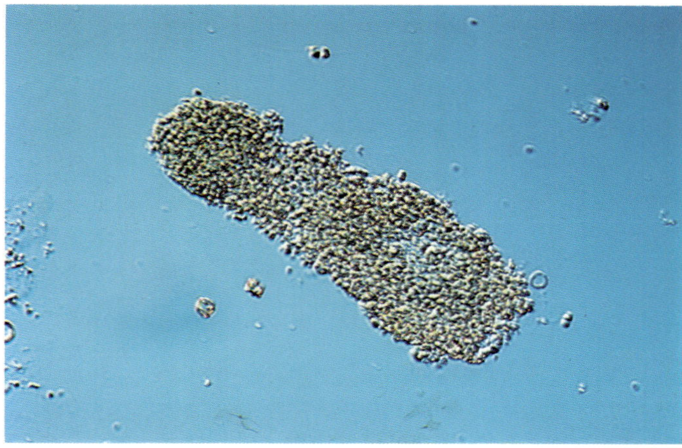

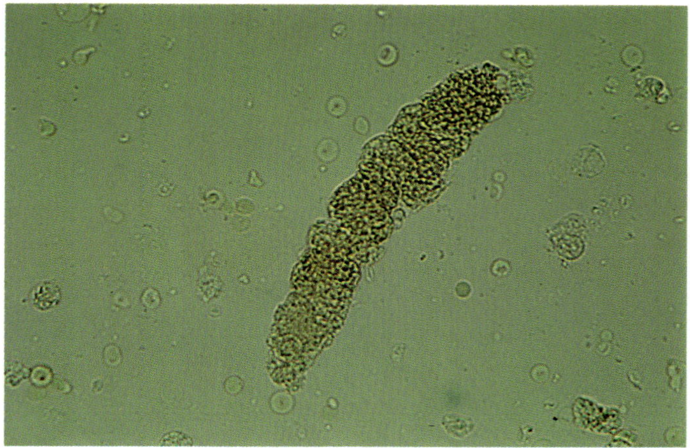

Fig 6–12. Granular cast, revealing certain cellular parts. Note numerous red cells and occasional white cells in the background (BF ×160).

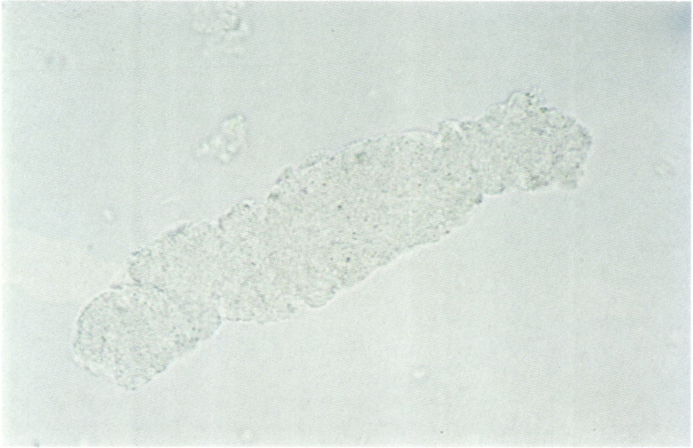

Fig 6–13. Broad, finely granular cast, in early stage of evolving into a waxy cast. Note notched margins and rather blunt ends (BF ×160).

Waxy Casts

Waxy casts are easily recognized by ordinary bright-field microscopy. They have a high refractive index, the highest of any cast, and are characterized by blunt or "broken-off" ends. Their margins are parallel and often show serrations, notches, or indentations, but may sometimes be smooth. They may be colorless or may have a yellowish, tan, or pale yellow and waxy appearance. Waxy casts are often broad and stubby, rather than narrow and elongated (Figs 6–14 and 6–15).

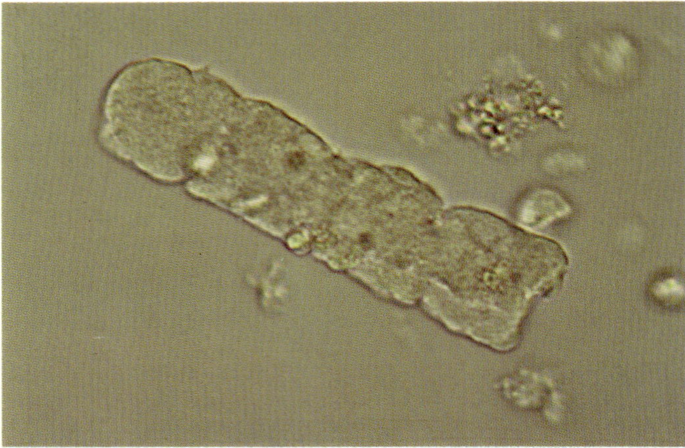

Fig 6–14. Typical waxy cast. Refractive index is high, ends are "broken-off," and parallel margins are irregular or serrated (BF ×250).

Because of their high refractivity, waxy casts are among the most easily seen and identified elements of the urinary sediment. They are not present in normal urine but are frequent accompaniments of the sediment in patients with intrinsic renal disease, especially the chronic varieties. The "broken-off" appearance of the ends is probably due to the fact that these casts are of relatively high density and therefore more fragile or brittle than other types. Waxy casts are thought to arise from preexistent cellular casts in which the intrinsic cellular components have broken down and degenerated into a relatively amorphous but "hard-appearing," featureless coating. Scanning electron miscroscopic techniques have shown that the surface

Fig 6–15. Same waxy cast depicted in Figure 6–14, but seen by phase-contrast microscopy. It appears much thicker than other casts, and its surface is somewhat granular (PH ×250).

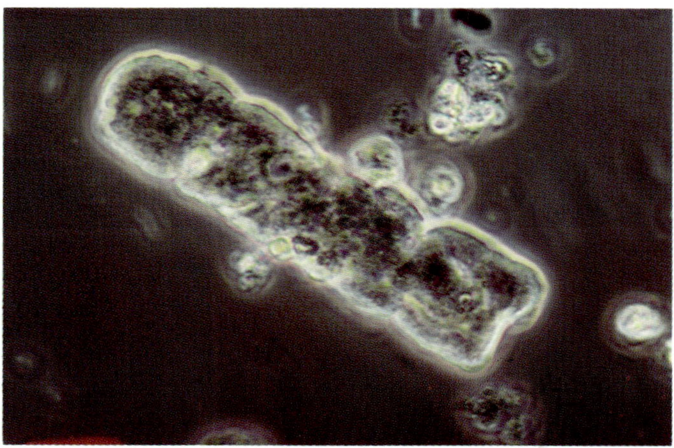

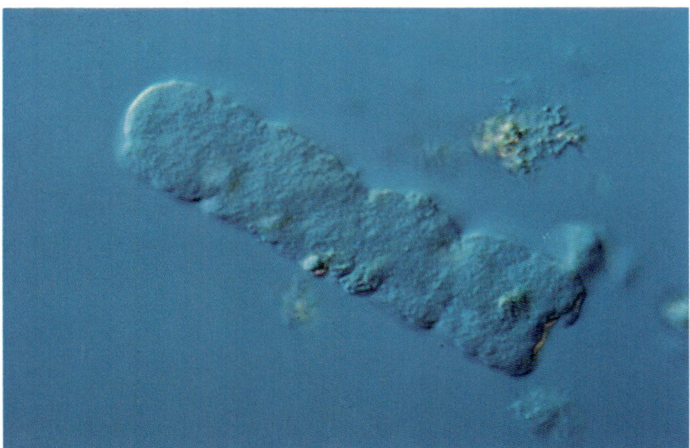

Fig 6–16. Waxy cast. Its particular waxy or platelike surface structure is easy to discern (ICM ×250).

of waxy casts has a "boiler plate" hard appearance composed of high-density granular material that may, at least in part, be cellular in origin.[22] However, the origin of waxy casts is not clearly established and remains in considerable doubt (Figs 6–16 and 6–17).

Clinically, the presence of waxy casts in the urine usually denotes renal disease of a relatively severe or progressive type. They are most often present in association with chronic glomerulonephritis, diabetic nephrosclerosis, malignant hypertension, and renal amyloidosis. They may be present in various forms of acute renal disease, but in these instances are seen less frequently and mostly in small numbers.

Fig 6–17. Waxy cast, typified by "broken-off" ends and parallel serrated margins. Its brittleness is apparent, as it appears to be "splitting" (Sternheimer-Malbin stain ×160).

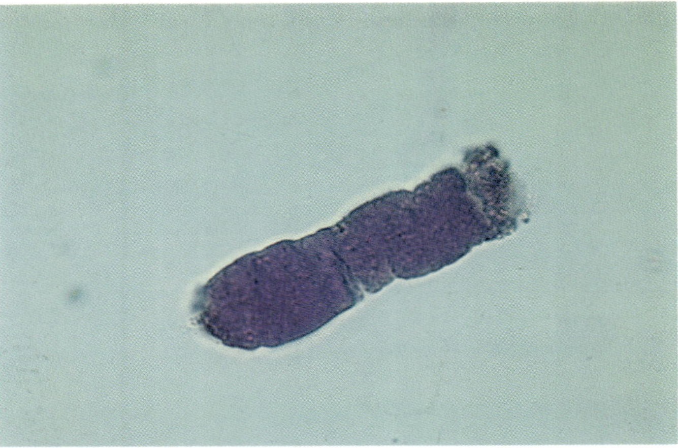

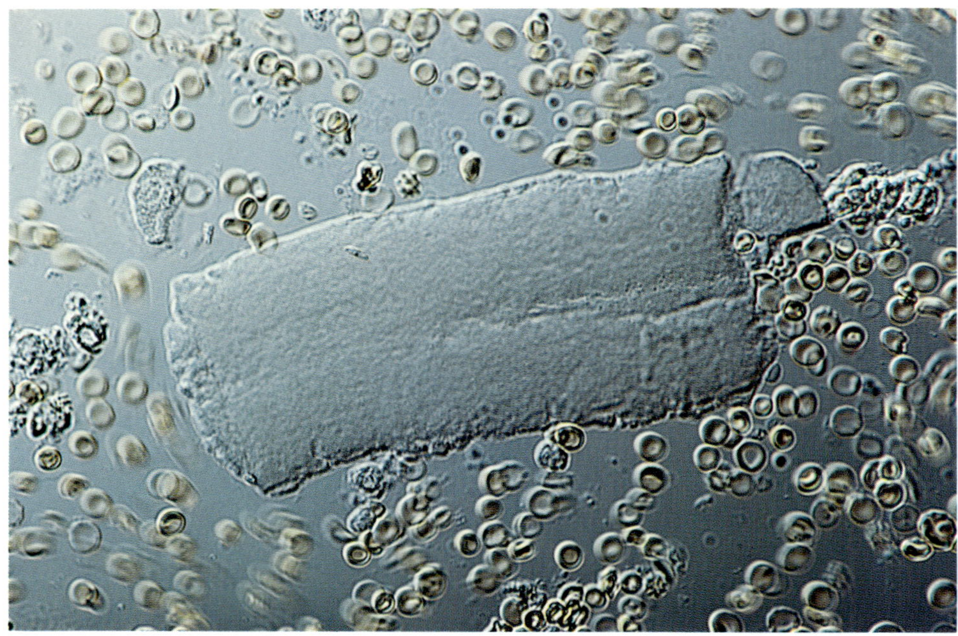

Fig 6–18. Waxy cast in urine with high refractive index, surrounded by abnormal sediment containing several PMNs and RBCs. Three-dimensional image is prototypic of casts except for unnotched sides (ICM ×160).

Waxy casts may be narrow or broad. As with other casts, a broad configuration usually denotes a relatively severe renal abnormality in which the nephrons are compromised to the extent that their lumina are dilated.[35] Waxy casts are not seen in large numbers in most diseases, irrespective of the severity or type of the disease. Their presence in the urine usually indicates a relatively long renal transit time, sufficient to produce molding and hardness.

The physical characteristics of waxy casts are readily recognized by any form of microscopy. The knobby indentations of their margins and their hard or brittle consistency are accentuated when either phase- or interference-contrast microscopy is used (Fig 6–18). This is in marked contrast to other types of casts, such as hyaline, in which the matrix is delicate and fibrillar and the margins are smooth. The crusty surface of waxy casts is unique and of major interest when studied with the scanning electron microscope.[22] Waxy casts rarely contain any cellular constituents recognizable as such but may include lipid globules on the surface (Fig 6–19).

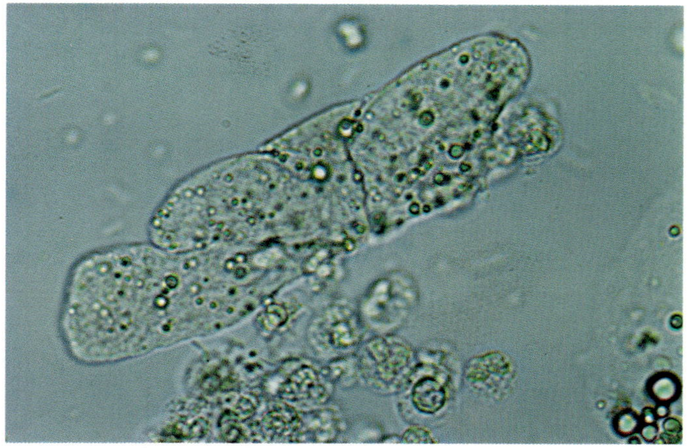

Fig 6–19. Broad waxy cast with notched margins and blunt ends, somewhat different from those previously illustrated. Note spheric lipid globules on its surface and numerous leukocytes in the background (BF ×250).

Fatty Casts

Fatty casts are casts that contain either free fat or oval fat bodies in which lipid is visibly apparent. Only those containing free fat will be discussed here. Many casts have a surface completely composed of lipid globules of varying shape and size. In other fatty casts the amount of lipid within or on the cast matrix is not as solidly packed and may be sparse.

Fatty casts are easily recognized microscopically (Figs 6–20 through 6–25), because they are composed of globular lipids and are yellowish tan. The lipids have a high refractive index, vary greatly in size and shape, and are birefringent. Under polarized microscopy these neutral fats appear in a "Maltese-cross" pattern. (The term "Maltese cross," when applied to the visualization of urinary fat is incorrect, although it is commonly used in medical parlance. In actual fact, a real Maltese cross has a different crossed pattern from that seen when anisotropic lipids are visualized under polarized light conditions.)[25]

The microscopist will often not be aware that the urine contains fat unless all abnormal urinary sediments are routinely polarized.[21] This takes only a few moments of time when using a microscope equipped with sliding polarizing prisms.

A word of caution needs to be interjected about the diagnosis of elements in the urinary sediment exhibiting anisotropism. Not all substances with these physical properties are lipids. In fact, a much more frequently observed finding is the birefringence displayed by many urinary crystals, especially urates. The observer must be careful when diagnosing lipid in the urine and should use all methods available, including polarized light, selective staining with sudanophilic dyes and, if necessary, chemical analysis before making a positive identification of fat in the urine.

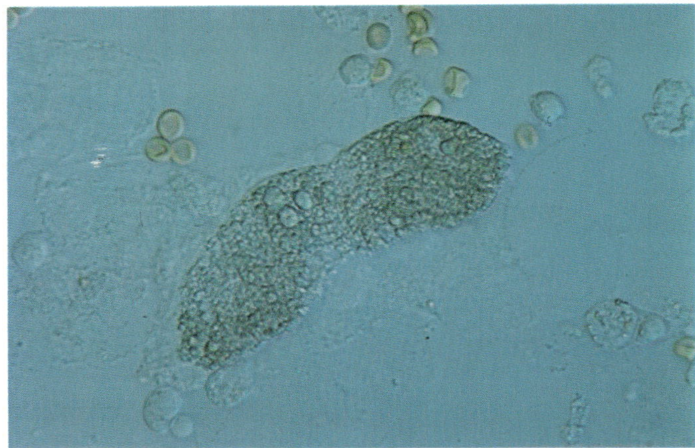

Fig 6–20. Typical fatty cast in urine. Entire surface seems to comprise lipid globules of variable sizes. In the background are several red cells and considerable cellular debris (BF ×200).

Fig 6–21. Polarization of fatty cast, same as shown in Figure 6–20. Note typical "Maltese-cross" pattern in larger lipid globules (Pol ×200).

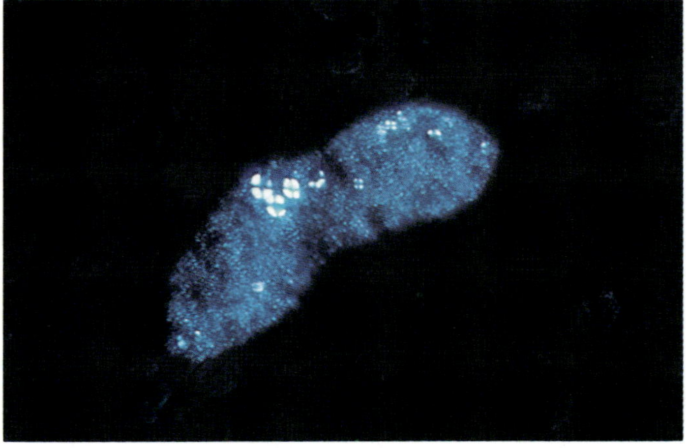

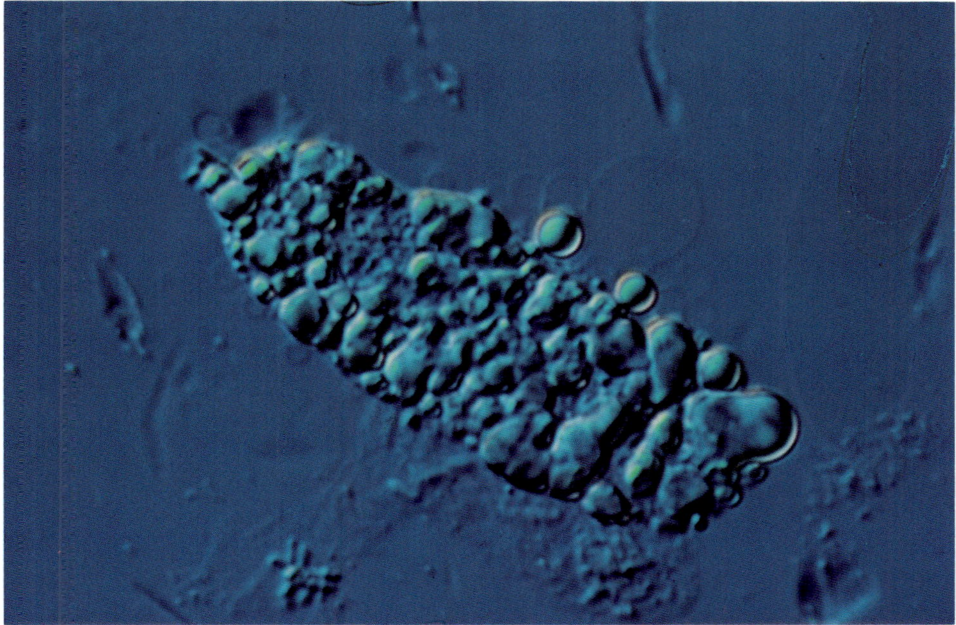

Fig 6–22. Fatty cast. Lipid globules are prominent on its surface, but some uninvolved surface areas can also be seen underlying the lipids. Some lipid globules are also adjacent to the cast (ICM ×400).

Pigmented Casts

A separate classification for this type of cast would ordinarily not be necessary. However, some explanation as to the presence of casts in the urine that contain adsorbed pigments or salts such as hemoglobin and bile is worth including. Basically, when large quantities of pigment are present in the urine in abnormal conditions, such as obstruction of the biliary tract or hemolytic anemia, bile or hemoglobin may be adsorbed into a hyaline matrix. The formerly transparent cast is then transformed into a colored one that is either yellow from bile or brownish red from hemoglobin (Fig 6–26). These casts may be specifically identified on the basis of their adsorbed product by appropriate chemical methods of analysis or by specific staining techniques (eg, hemoglobin). Bile casts are often accompanied in the urine by large numbers of renal epithelial cells or epithelial casts, or both, and are chemically associated with the presence of large quantities of bilirubin or urobilinogen, or both. Hemoglobin casts, on the other hand, are classically present in severe hemolytic anemia or in other diseases that produce marked hemolysis. In such instances large quantities of hemoglobin or its by-products are filtered through the glomerulus and thus appear in the urine.

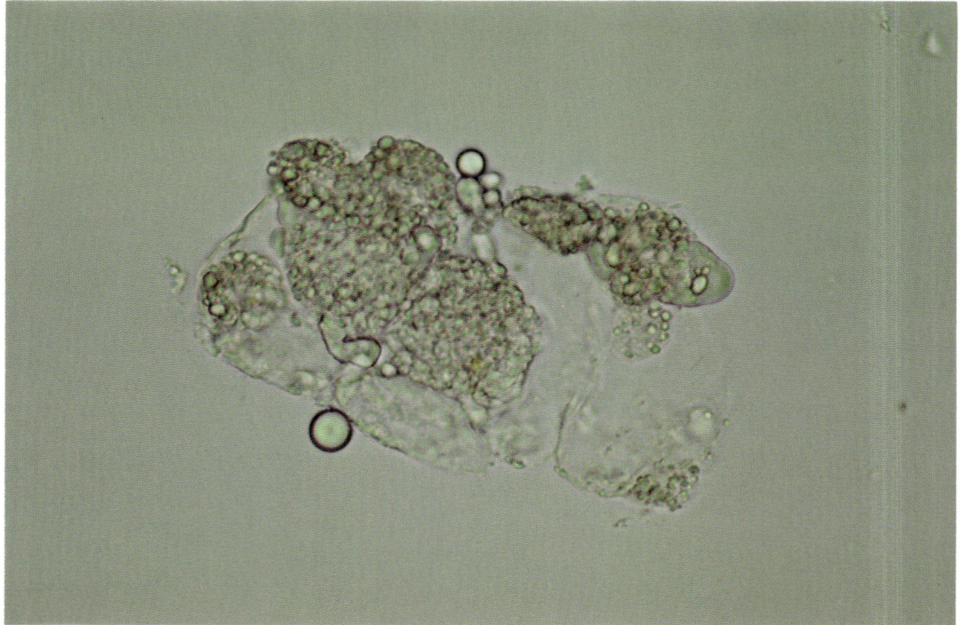

Fig 6–23. Mixed cast (waxy and fatty) with fat globules and granules superimposed. The lipids are highly refractile, globular, and varying greatly as to size and shape. Some free-floating fat globules are also adjacent to the cast (BF ×160).

Fig 6–24. Mixed cast (waxy and fatty), showing birefringence and classic "Maltese-cross" features of urinary lipids, within the cast and adjacent fat globules (Pol ×160).

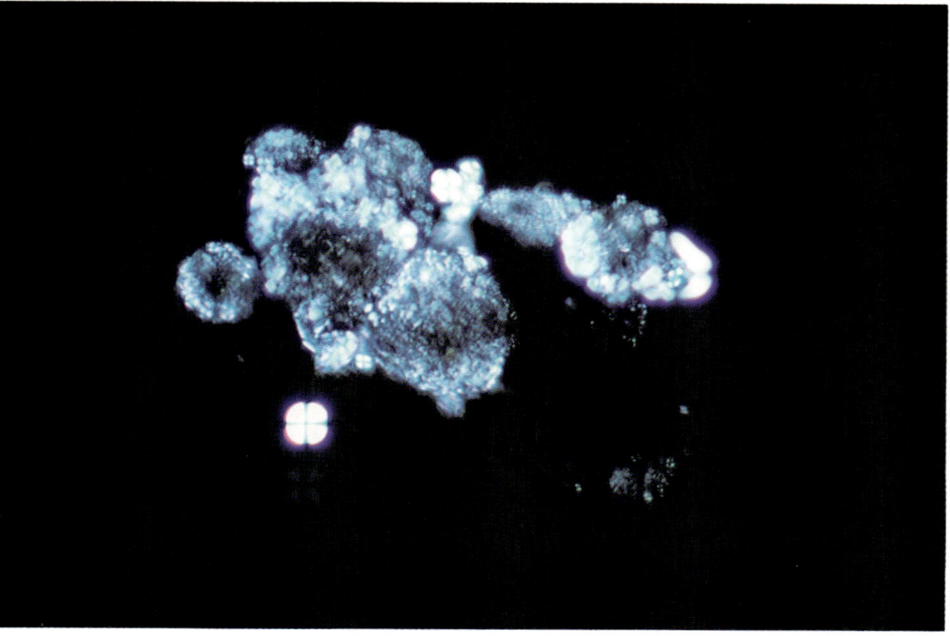

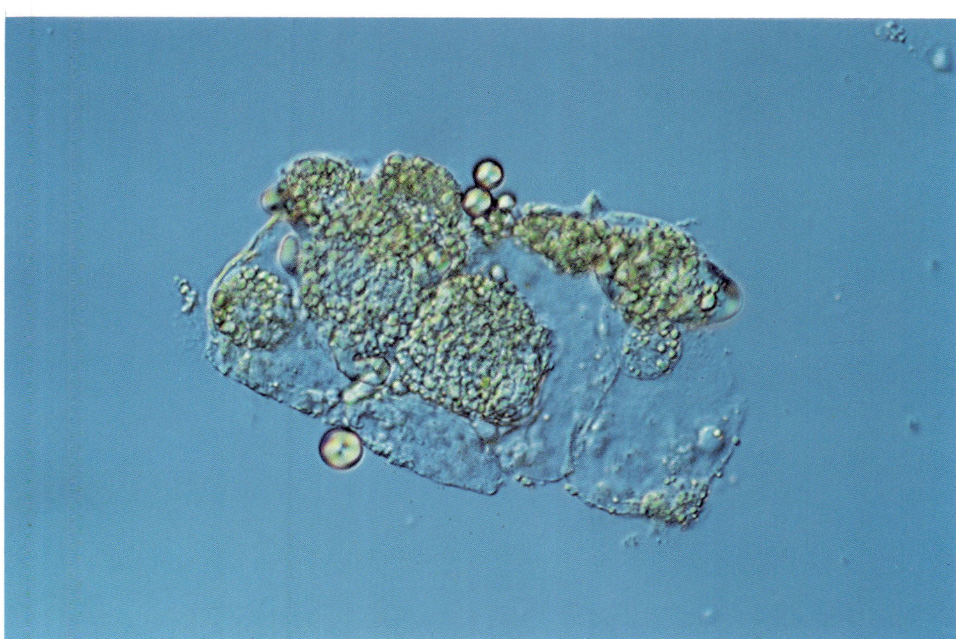

Fig 6–25. Mixed cast (waxy and fatty), identical to Figures 6–23 and 6–24, but visualized with interference-contrast microscopy. Lipids are yellowish, three-dimensional, spheric globules. Sharply outlined cast has squared-off ends and irregular margins, indicating waxy nature (ICM ×160).

Other pigmented casts, such as those present in patients with renal amyloidosis or multiple myeloma (Bence Jones protein), are rare and may be difficult to identify because of the fact that the material comprising or adsorbed into the cast matrix is not colored. However, chemical analysis or specific staining will reveal the true composition of these casts.

Fig 6–26. Histologic section of pigmented bile casts forming in renal tubule from case of viral hepatitis where bile pigment was heavily concentrated in the urine (H&E ×160).

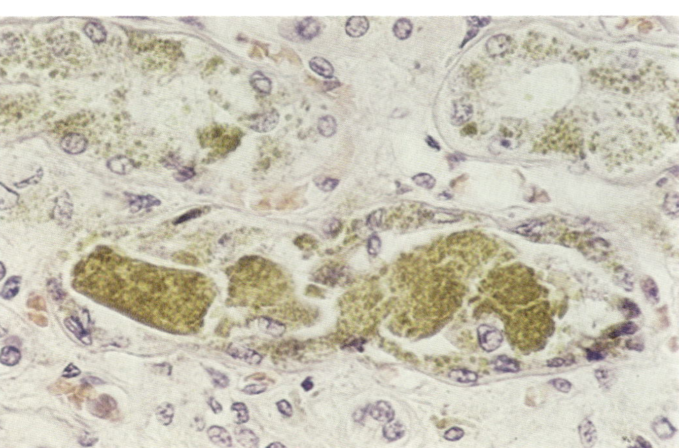

CELLULAR CASTS

Nearly all casts form primarily in the distal tubule and collecting duct portions of the nephron. Since this is the case, it is self-evident that casts are unique to the kidney and are not formed elsewhere in the urinary tract. For this reason, the presence of casts in the urine has special clinical significance, and if abnormal cast forms are seen, the disease of which they are a manifestation concentrates the pathologic process specifically within the kidney, rather than any other part of the urinary tract.

All casts have a common hyaline matrix composed of fibrillar proteinaceous material, a part of which is a Tamm-Horsfall protein.[22] Depending on the type and cause of damage to the nephron, and the location and duration of injury, various types of cells may leak or be sloughed into the urinary stream and become incorporated into a cast (Fig 6–27).

Cellular casts are named from and may be diagnosed on the basis of the type of cells they are composed of, ie, blood cells (RBC or WBC), epithelial cells, or bacteria. Cellular casts are not normally found in the urinary sediment. Thus, when they are observed, they indicate a pathologic state in the patient, most often an intrinsic renal disease.[51, 52] Since only two blood cell types are commonly seen in the urinary sediment, namely, erythrocytes and leukocytes, casts containing substantial numbers of these cells are designated accordingly, eg, *red blood cell casts* or *white blood cell casts*. Renal epithelial cells, on the other hand, are not morphologically similar in all parts of the nephron but vary depending on the specific portion from which they originate (ie, proximal tubular cell, Henle cell). However, for practical purposes, renal epithelial cells are lumped together and considered similar when found in the urine, and casts containing these cells are called *epithelial casts*.

Fig 6–27. Mechanisms of cellular cast formation in the nephron. (From Haber.[20] Used by permission.)

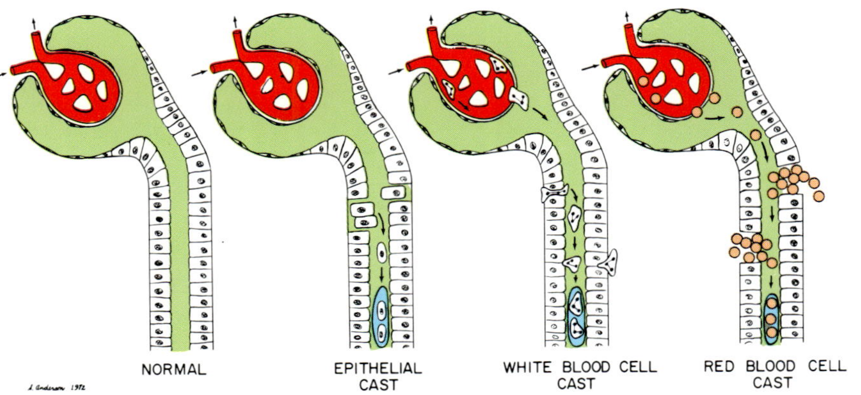

Recently, in our own laboratory, we have found a third type of cellular cast in the urine of patients with pyelonephritis.[37] This cast, the *bacterial cast*, has as a major component unicellular microorganisms. We have only seen bacterial casts in patients with pyelonephritis, and they will be discussed at length later in this chapter.

Cells within a cast often undergo degeneration during their transit through the kidney and the lower urinary tract. This results in cellular breakdown, loss of cell membranes, degeneration, pyknosis, karyolysis of the nuclei, and the formation of granular or amorphous material, which may be observed as debris in a granular cast. It thus is certain that in many instances where pathologic states exist, granular casts are formed as a direct result of the degeneration of preexistent cellular casts (see Fig 6–1).

When the prototype cast is composed of red blood cells, breakdown and dissolution of the erythrocytes result in what is commonly called a *blood cast*. Breakdown of either epithelial or white blood cells in their respective casts may result in the production of granular casts that appear similar and cannot be distinguished from one another. Granular casts may similarly undergo an evolution during their transit through the nephron and evolve into what we presently designate as *waxy casts*. The morphologic alterations resulting in this evolution are thought to involve the coagulation of cellular protein into a thick, crusty surface substance that is highly refractile and appears waxy when observed under light microscopy.

Cellular casts may be either narrow or broad. As we have seen, broadness in a cast suggests permanent degeneration of the nephron from which it came. That is, broad casts are formed in dilated distal tubules or collecting ducts. When large numbers of broad casts are in the urine, this is therefore considered a poor prognostic sign.

Red Blood Cell Casts

Red blood cell casts (erythrocyte or RBC casts) are perhaps the most diagnostically significant of all elements found in the urinary sediment.[51] Although red blood cells may enter the urinary stream via disrupted tubular elements, their most common means of entry is through a damaged glomerular basement membrane. The presence of many red blood cell casts in the urinary sediment is therefore ordinarily considered an indicator of glomerular injury.[24, 28] These casts are most often found in the urine in diseases such as glomerulonephritis, lupus nephritis, Goodpasture's syndrome, subacute bacterial endocarditis, and focal glomerulitis.[63] However, other renal diseases that may or may not cause direct damage to or destroy the glomerulus give rise to red blood cell casts and hematuria. The more common of these include acute pyelonephritis and renal infarction.[21]

A glomerular basement membrane injury giving rise to red cells in the urine must be sufficiently severe to allow erythrocytes from the bloodstream to enter the urinary flow with facility. Once in Bowman's space as a component of the glomerular filtrate and then in the tubular lumen, these red cells are attached to the surface of a hyaline cast matrix. Scanning electron microscopic studies have demonstrated thin proteinaceous fibrils (possibly fibrin, in part) attaching erythrocytes to the cast matrix in a complex and efficient manner.

Red blood cell casts are recognized in the urine sediment with relative ease. The erythrocytes often maintain their biconcave disc shape, and contained hemoglobin appears tan or brown (Figs 6–28 and 6–29). One may observe crenated erythrocytes on occasion in certain casts. It is often asked how many red cells must be present in a given cast for one to diagnose it as a red blood cell cast. This question is not easily answered. Suffice it to say that more than one or two red cells are necessary. A general rule of thumb in cast diagnosis is that at least one third or more of the cast surface should be composed of the specific cell type for the cast to be named accordingly.

Erythrocyte casts evolve as they pass through the nephron. The red cells may lose their cellular membranes and degenerate, thus allowing hemoglobin to leak out of the cell and into the surrounding cast matrix (Figs 6–30 and 6–31). These degenerative changes result in blood casts. Evidence that such a cast arose from a preexistent red blood cell cast is established by identifying red cell membranes in the cast and noting the peculiar reddish orange color resulting from hemoglobin pigment leaking into the cast matrix.

Interference-contrast and phase-contrast microscopy enable the observer to diagnose RBC casts more readily, as does sediment staining with Sternheimer-Malbin dyes (Fig 6–32).[6, 57] Red cells may be densely or loosely packed in the cast. This feature of erythrocyte density within the cast is considered by some to be an indicator of how severe the transglomerular bleeding that caused the cast formation was. Blood casts may be somewhat more difficult to identify, since they contain few erythrocyte remnants (Fig 6–33).

Fig 6–28. Red blood cell cast. Erythrocytes are more densely concentrated towards one end of hyaline cast matrix (BF ×160).

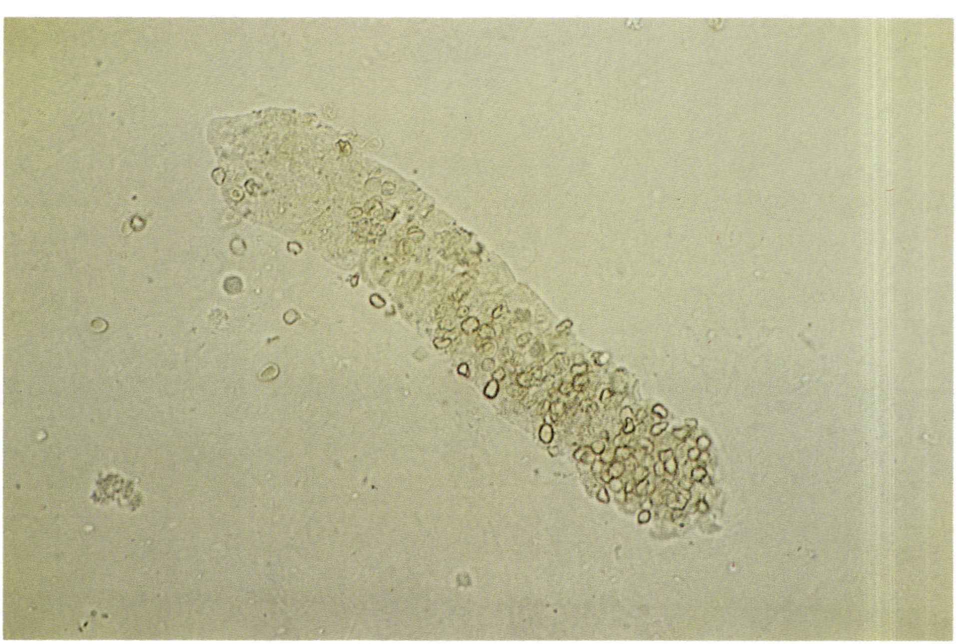

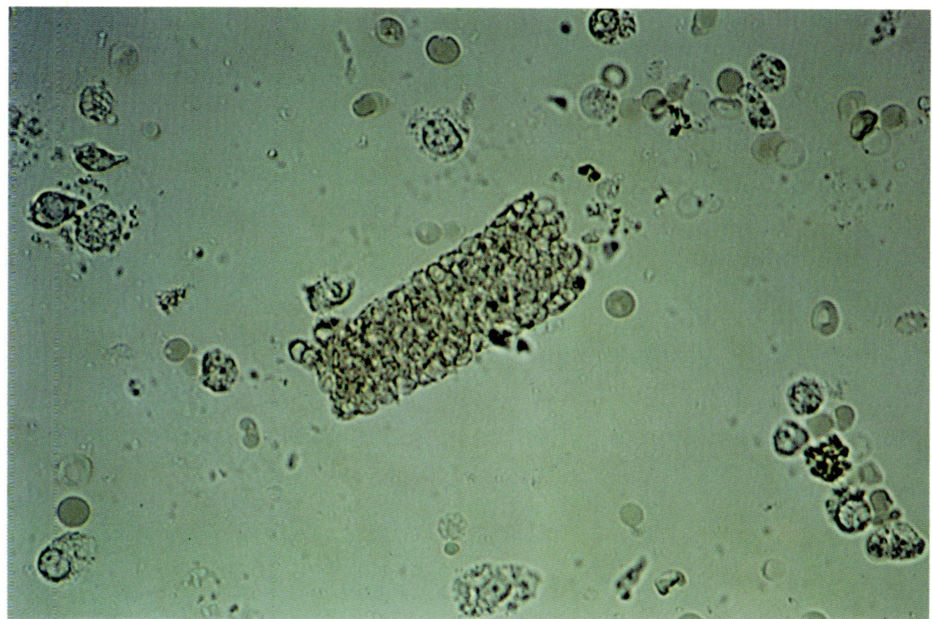

Fig 6–29. Red blood cell cast, showing predominantly intact erythrocytes closely packed together. Surrounding urine is filled with numerous PMNs and erythrocytes (BF ×160).

Fig 6–30. Red blood cell and hemoglobin cast. Erythrocytes have degenerated, resulting in granular, yellowish brown hemoglobin in the cast matrix. However, numerous intact erythrocytes are still present and easily identifiable on the surface (ICM ×200).

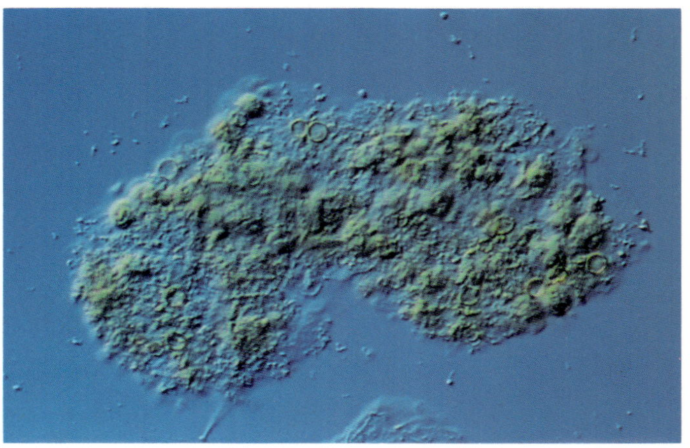

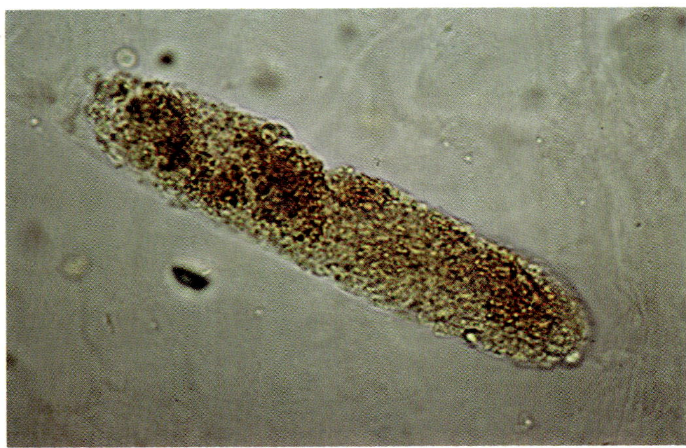

Fig 6–31. Red blood cell and hemoglobin cast, almost entirely composed of granular hemoglobin material. Remnants of erythrocyte cell walls can occasionally be seen (BF ×200).

Fig 6–32. Red blood cell hemoglobin cast, predominantly including purplish-dyed, granular hemoglobin. Erythrocytic components are primarily disrupted, though some cell walls and intact RBCs remain in the background (Sternheimer-Malbin stain ×200).

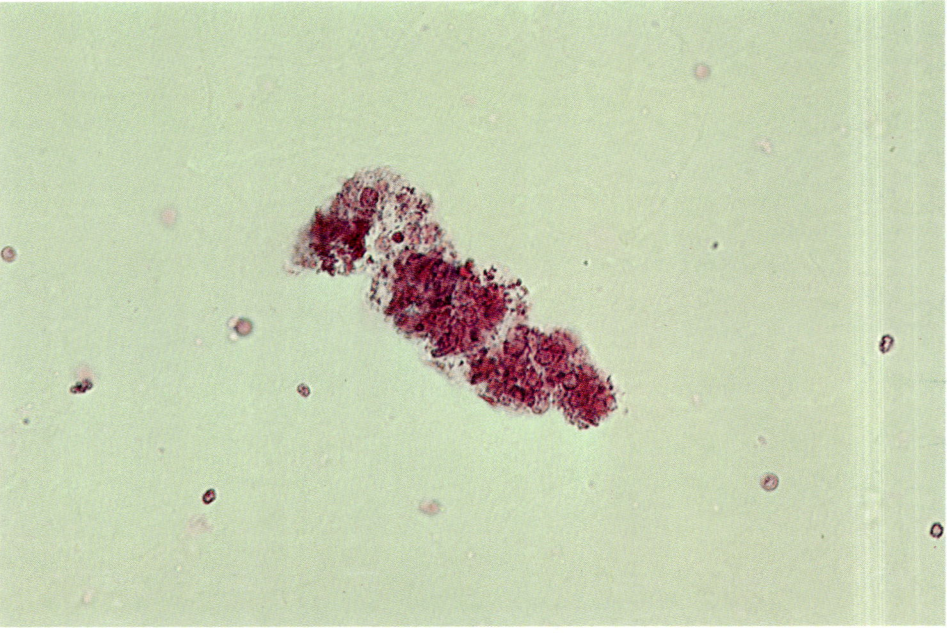

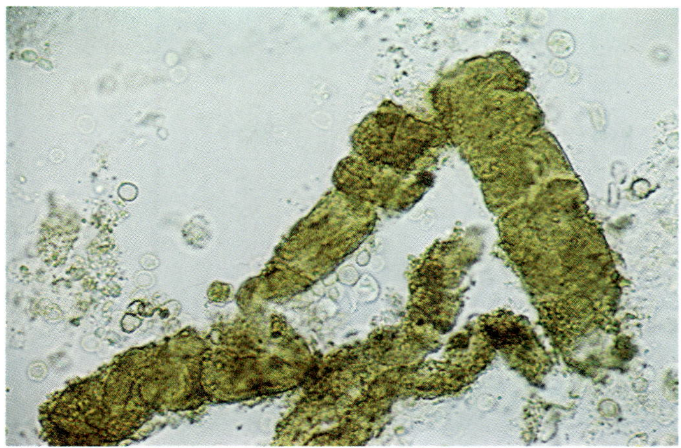

Fig 6–33. Hemoglobin casts, surrounded by abnormal erythrocytes and leukocytes. Casts vary greatly in size and shape, have a high refractive index, and are brownish tan, with practically no intact erythrocytes (BF ×160).

White Blood Cell Casts

White blood cell casts (WBC or leukocyte casts) are identified with relative ease in the urine sediment. They are not present in normal urinary specimens, and therefore when discovered are considered a pathologic finding. Their presence in the urine is most often associated with kidney infections. However, these casts are frequently seen in many other types of intrinsic renal disease, especially diseases in which an inflammatory component involving the kidney is present. White blood cells incorporated into these casts enter the urinary stream by either of two major pathways—transglomerular or transtubular (see Fig 6–27). In inflammations of the kidney in which an interstitial component predominates, as in acute pyelonephritis, the white cells (mostly PMNs) move by ameboid motion through the tubular basement membrane, between renal epithelial cells lining the tubular portions of the nephron, and into the lumen of the tubule.[24] This transtubular mechanism seems to predominate in intrinsic renal infections. However, the second mechanism by which WBCs enter the urinary flow—transglomerular—is also of considerable importance, especially in other renal diseases that produce a significant inflammatory component, such as lupus nephritis, polyarteritis nodosa, and acute glomerulonephritis. In these instances, white cells migrate from the bloodstream across the glomerular basement membrane and into Bowman's space as a component of the glomerular filtrate. It is obvious that in both of these mechanisms, proteinuria is almost invariably associated with the leukouria. In addition, when bacterial infections of the kidney initiate the inflammatory response, bacteriuria is also seen.

The clinical differentiation of primary diseases involving the interstitial tissues of the kidney, such as pyelonephritis, from immunologic diseases involving the glomerulus or tubular structures of the nephron is sometimes difficult and cannot ordinarily be made purely from the presence of leukocyte casts in the urine. In such instances, a carefully taken clinical history in conjunction with certain laboratory tests will help to illuminate the diagnosis. Pyelonephritis is often manifested clinically by flank pain and fever.[10] On the other hand, immunologic diseases such as glomerulonephritis are often preceded by an upper respiratory infection and are accompanied by different urinary sediment findings such as large numbers of red blood cell casts.

A pathognomonic urinary sediment finding that, in our experience, has been confined exclusively to patients with intrinsic renal infection (ie, pyelonephritis) is the presence of bacterial casts.[37] We have observed that bacteria are incorporated into the cast structure, often along with white blood cells, in this disease entity.

From this brief summary, it is readily apparent that white blood cell casts in the urine are not diagnostic of a single disease entity and may be present in association with a variety of renal abnormalities. White cell casts are often accompanied in the sediment by a wide range of many of the other casts discussed in this chapter; among the most frequent are hyaline and granular casts.

The recognition of white blood cell casts in the urine is ordinarily not difficult. The leukocytes themselves, when preserved intact on the cast matrix, appear as neutrophils in the peripheral blood.[58] They are usually, but not always, PMNs (Figs 6–34 through 6–38). However, mononuclear white blood cells, such as lymphocytes and monocytes, may also be seen, but infrequently. Neutrophils measure 15–20 μ in greatest diameter and have granules in their cytoplasm. Neutrophilic nuclei are multilobed and stain with basic dyes. The PMNs in casts often show visible

Fig 6–34. White blood cell cast in which leukocytes are intact and easily identified as having multilobed nuclei. In some areas, hyaline matrix can still be seen and is not obscured by heavy concentration of PMNs (BF ×160).

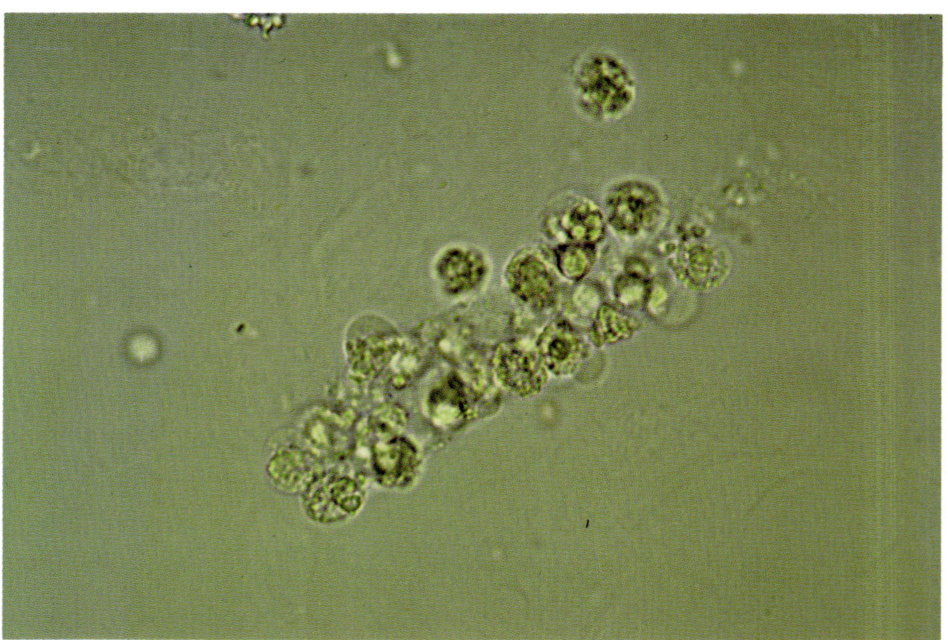

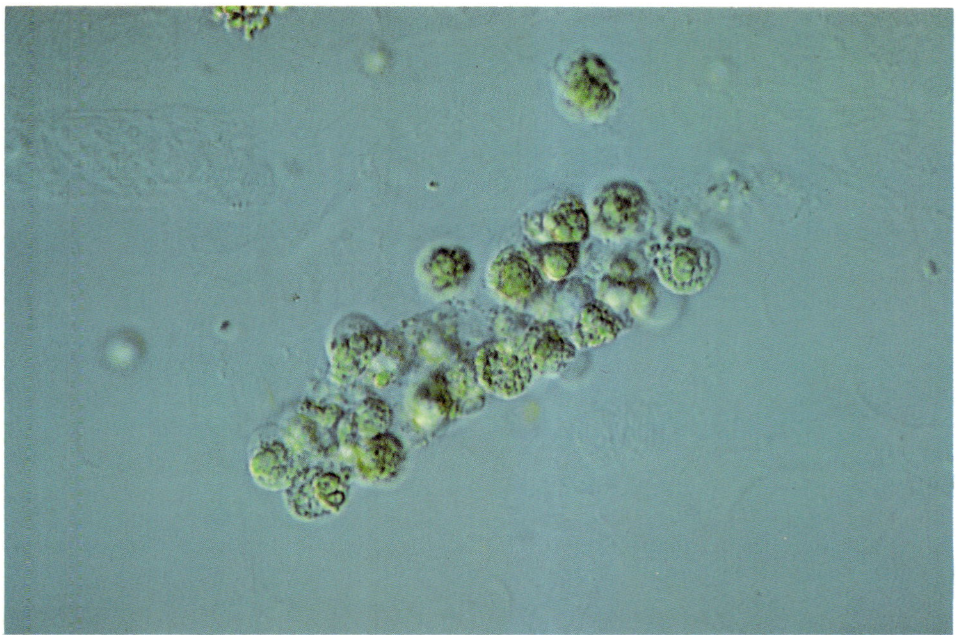

Fig 6–35. Same white blood cell cast as in Figure 6–34, now shown under interference-contrast microscopy. Characteristic features are more prominent than previously, and hyaline nature of matrix is readily displayed (ICM ×160).

Fig 6–36. Histologic section of white cell cast in renal tubule lumen. Hyaline matrix is the basis of a cast in which leukocytes are packed into a segment (H&E ×100).

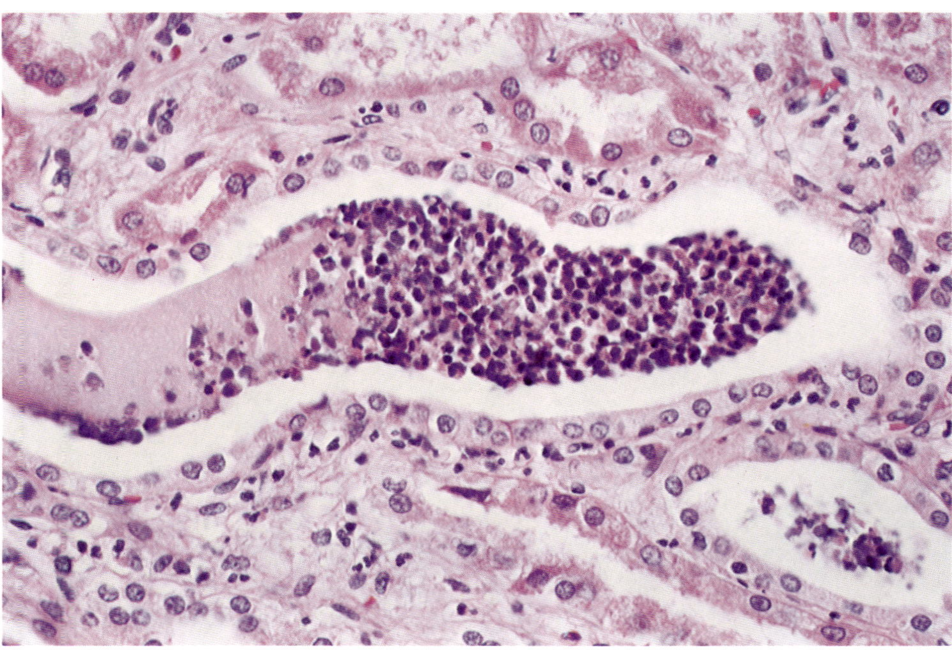

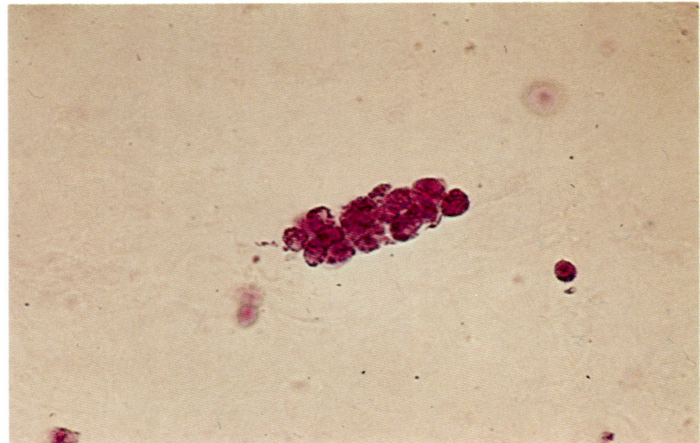

Fig 6–37. White blood cell cast, easily identified as cellular in nature. Component cells are spheric, intact, and have granular cytoplasm; their nuclei are difficult to discern (Sternheimer-Malbin stain ×160).

signs of degeneration and commonly appear as disrupted cells with indistinct cell membranes and multifragmented nuclei. Eosinophils or basophils are rarely seen incorporated into casts.

Interference-contrast microscopy is particularly helpful in the recognition of WBC casts. This microscopic technique enables the observer to visualize the multilobed leukocytic nuclei with greater facility (as does staining), which is often helpful in specific cast diagnosis, since many of the WBCs show degenerative signs (Fig 6–39).[18, 57]

Fig 6–38. White cell cast, displaying multilobed characteristics of neutrophils. Hyaline matrix can be seen in certain areas. One or two neutrophils are beginning to degenerate with nuclear disappearance and disruption of cell membranes (BF ×250).

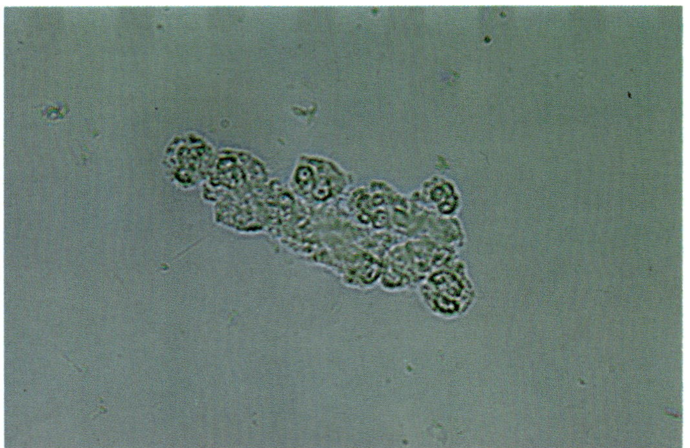

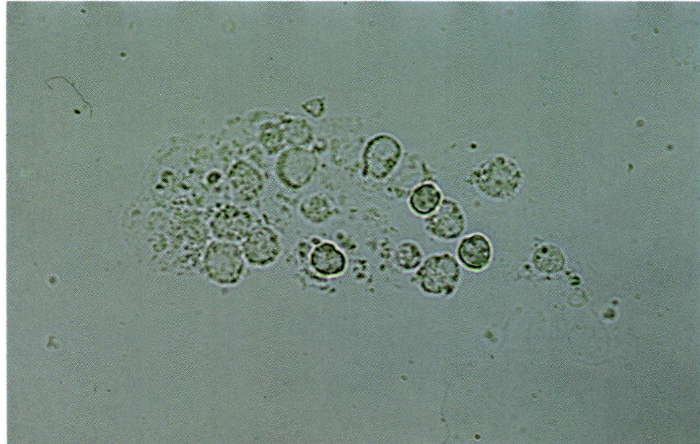

Fig 6–39. White blood cell cast, showing marked degeneration. Most leukocytes are difficult to identify due to disrupted cell walls and nondistinct nuclei. The cells are attached to the hyaline matrix surface (BF ×200).

White blood cell casts may be confused with epithelial casts, since these cells are of similar size. Epithelial cells, however, have large single nuclei. In addition, the cytoplasm of the PMN is granular and comprises a much greater proportion of the cell volume than does the cytoplasm of the epithelial cell.

Epithelial Casts

Epithelial cells in the urine derive their origin from renal tubular epithelium lining the nephron. As previously stated, this epithelium varies morphologically in each segment of the nephron.[55] In histologic sections of the kidney, specific portions of the nephron, and therefore the cells lining them, can be distinguished one from another with great facility. However, when these cells are present in the urine sediment, the distinction as to exactly what portion of the nephron they originate from is considerably less clear. In fact, it is often difficult to distinguish cells of renal epithelial origin from those lining the lower urinary tract, which are of transitional origin.

In diseases of the kidney in which tubules of the nephron are affected, epithelial cells are oftentimes sloughed into the urinary stream and become incorporated into a cast matrix (see Fig 6–27). Since casts form only in the kidney, one need only recognize cells of epithelial origin (as contrasted from leukocytes or red blood cells) within the cast to identify this type of cast specifically. As in the cellular casts previously discussed, the epithelial cells are bound to the cast surface by thin fibrillar proteinaceous strands.[22]

Epithelial casts are not present in the urine of healthy persons. These casts are easily recognized because of their high refractive index and epithelial cell component (Figs 6–40 through 6–42). Renal epithelial cells have large nuclei (approximately 10–12 μ in diameter) and a relatively sparse amount of agranular cytoplasm.

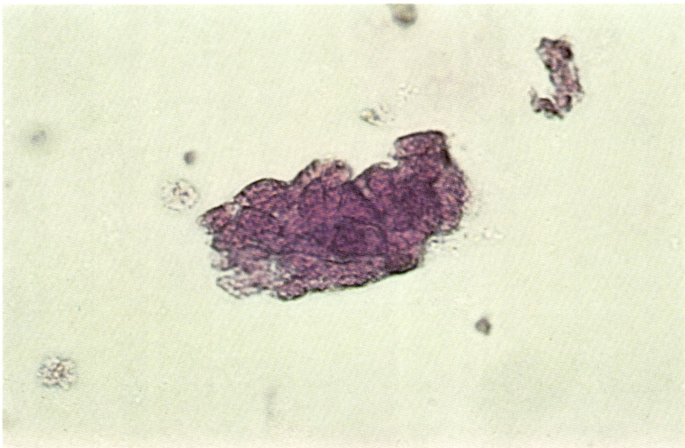

Fig 6–40. Epithelial cast, featuring large, polyhedral cells with central, spheric nuclei that are easily discerned (Sternheimer-Malbin stain ×200).

Fig 6–41. Epithelial cast. Several well circumscribed and intact tubular epithelial cells, imbedded in a hyaline cast matrix, are easily identified as to type (BF ×160).

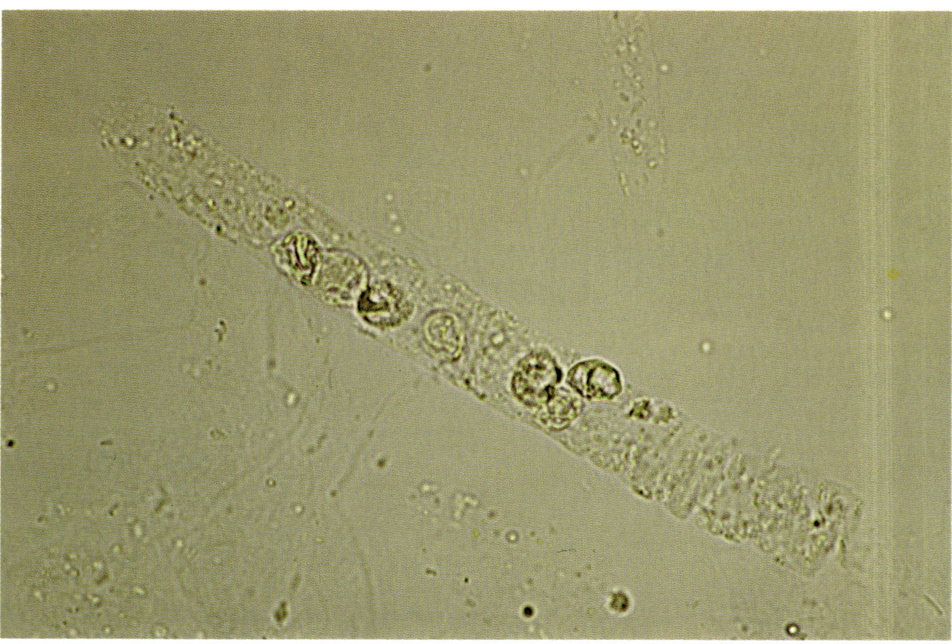

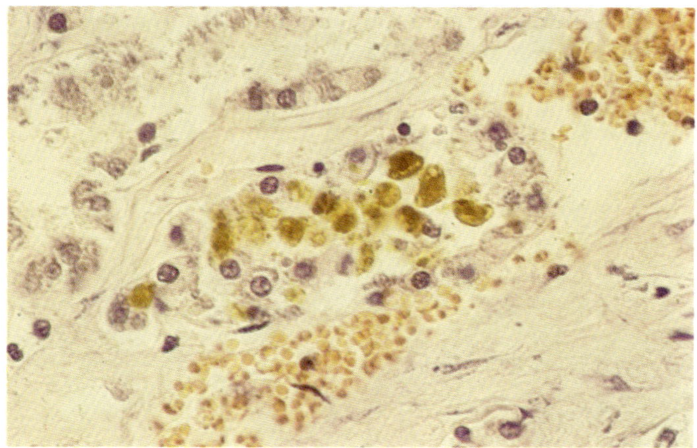

Fig 6–42. Histologic section of proximal renal tubule, showing numerous bile-stained epithelial cells, sloughed into the lumen and incorporated into hyaline cast matrix, forming epithelial casts. The cells are polyhedral and contain large, central, spheric nuclei. Bile pigmentation of the cytoplasm enhances their identification (H&E ×160).

The cell membrane is distinct, and the cells themselves often have a polyhedral, elongate, or columnar shape. However, some may appear cuboidal or flattened. Cells may be found in the casts either intact or in various stages of degeneration (Fig 6–43). When carefully examined, some renal epithelial cells may show a microvillous border along one end (ie, they are of proximal tubular origin). The epithelial cells in the cast may be organized in a relatively regular pattern and aligned

Fig 6–43. Epithelial cast. Large cells with central, spheric nuclei and granular hyaline matrix are visible (ICM ×250).

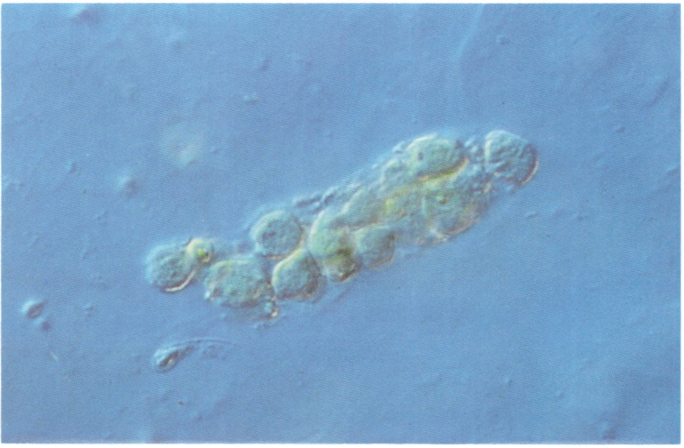

in rows along the length of the cast, or they may be totally disoriented from one another on the cast surface. When the cells are arranged in parallel rows, rather than haphazardly, this is thought to indicate damage to a specific localized segment of the nephron.[44, 63] This type of cast appearance is frequently associated with diseases in which a toxin has affected a given segment of the renal tubule and contiguous desquamation has occurred.

Epithelial cells present in these casts may undergo considerable degeneration during their transit through the nephron. When this occurs, cell and nuclear membranes disappear, and the granular products in the cytoplasm become incorporated into the cast matrix. Specific staining and the application of phase or interference contrast help the observer to identify these casts when significant degrees of degeneration have occurred.[18, 19]

Epithelial casts may be either broad or narrow. They are found in the urinary sediment in a wide variety of diseases involving the kidney but are especially prominent in the general category of diseases called the *nephroses*. In such instances, a specific ingested nephrotoxin, such as bichloride of mercury or diethylene glycol, may cause renal tubular epithelial cell damage.[14, 24, 51] More recently, epithelial casts have been noted in the urine of patients receiving chemotherapeutic agents for the treatment of malignant disease.[54] Many chemotherapeutic drugs are nephrotoxic and produce extensive cellular damage and epithelial sloughing, which result in formation of epithelial casts. A third major group of human diseases that commonly affect the renal tubular cell and result in the formation of epithelial casts are certain viral diseases such as hepatitis, and respiratory viral infectious agents such as cytomegalovirus (Figs 6–44 through 6–51). In such instances, the virus invades the renal tubular epithelial cell and causes its death. The cell subsequently sloughs into the urine. Diseases that involve extensive glomerular injury, and therefore secondary tubular disruption, may also produce this form of cast.

Fig 6–44. Epithelial cell cast. Note that the large, polyhedral renal tubular epithelial cells on the hyaline matrix contain considerable bile pigment and are easily identified. They are beginning to show degenerative changes (ICM ×200).

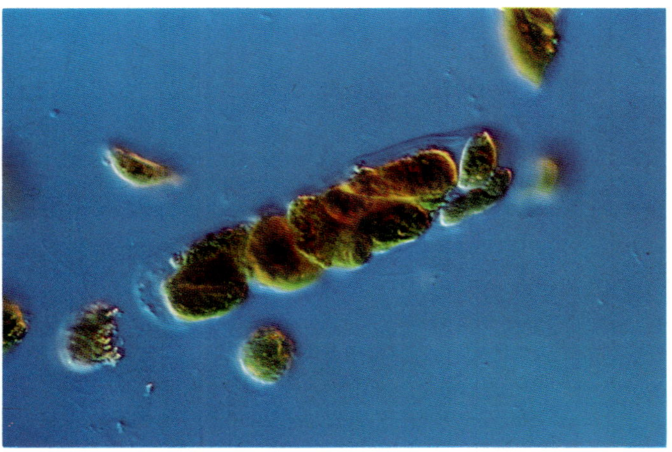

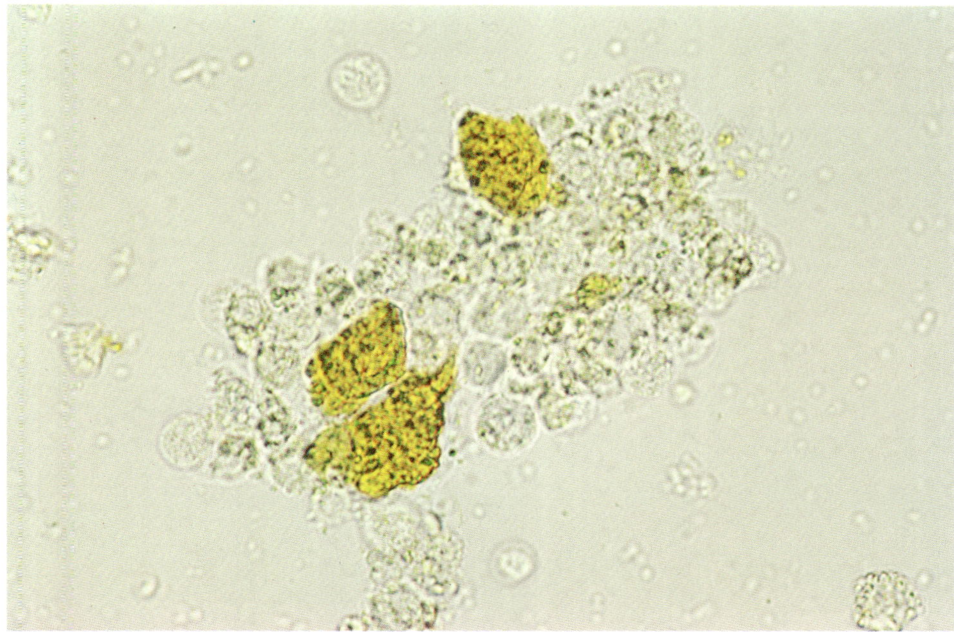

Fig 6–45. Mixed cast (epithelial and white cell). Epithelial cells are readily identified, since they are much larger than adjacent leukocytes and are bile stained; they are beginning to show some cytoplasmic and nuclear degeneration. The leukocytes are nearly transparent and also show some degeneration, but many cytoplasmic granules and multilobed nuclei are discernible (BF ×160).

Fig 6–46. Degenerating epithelial cast, evolving into a granular cast. In one epithelial cell, a nucleus with nucleolus is apparent. Remaining cells have granular cytoplasm and disrupted cell walls. In the cast matrix, numerous coarse granules can easily be seen (PH ×250).

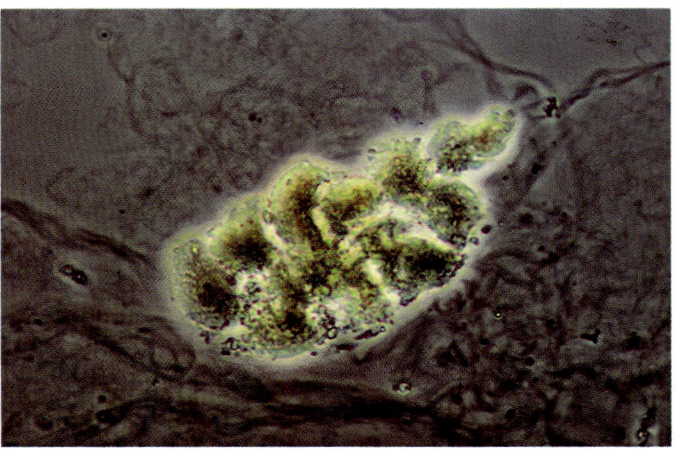

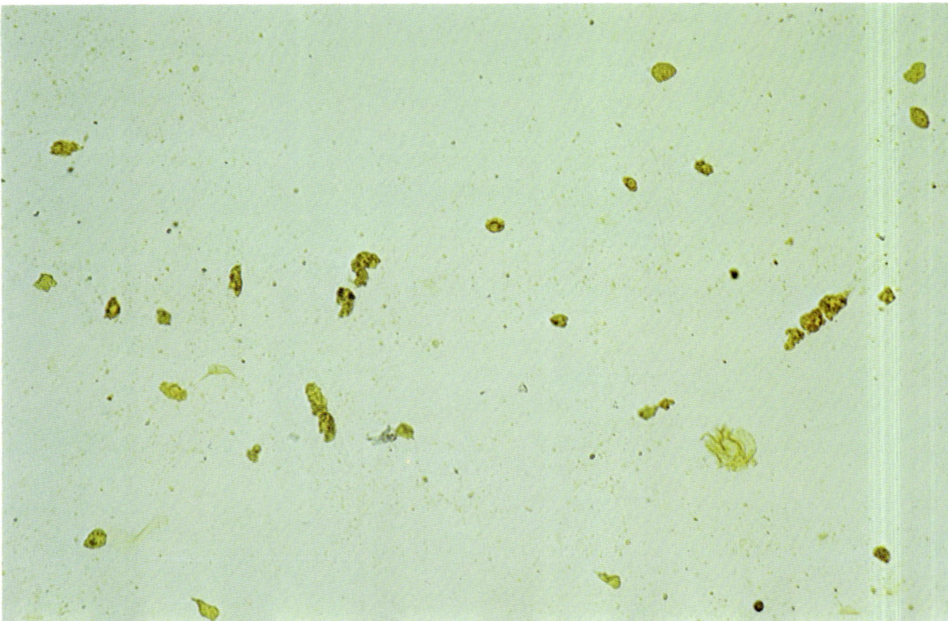

Fig 6–47. Epithelial casts in urine. This low-power view demonstrates the number of these casts that may be present in a severe viral disease involving the kidney, ie, viral hepatitis. The casts are easily seen, even at this power, since they contain pigmented epithelial cells (BF ×40).

Fig 6–48. Epithelial cast with a "tail," ie, cylindroid appearance. Surface cells show marked degeneration with cytoplasmic vacuolization and nuclear disruption. Cast matrix shows considerable granularity. In the background, numerous erythrocytes, cytoplasmic debris, and occasional leukocytes are present (BF ×200).

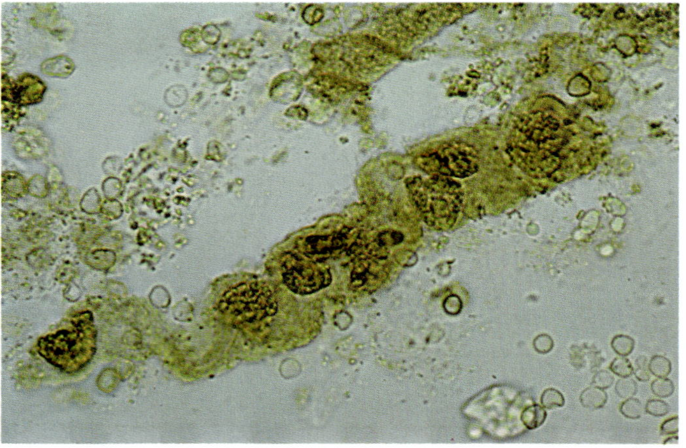

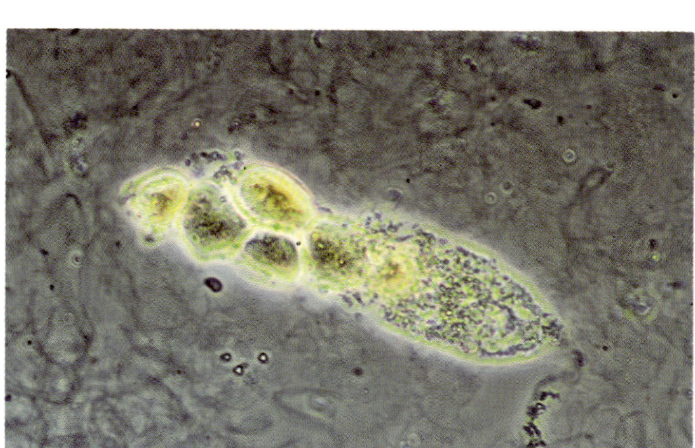

Fig 6–49. Mixed cast (epithelial and granular). Phase-contrast microscopy enhances matrix granularity. Epithelial cells are obvious at one end and show little cellular detail, since they are in varying stages of degeneration. Considerable fibrillar mucus is present in the background (PH ×250).

Fig 6–50. Mixed cast (epithelial and granular), same as shown in Figure 6–49. Interference-contrast microscopy greatly enhances morphologic features. Again, granularity at one end is in contrast to epithelial component at opposite end (ICM ×250).

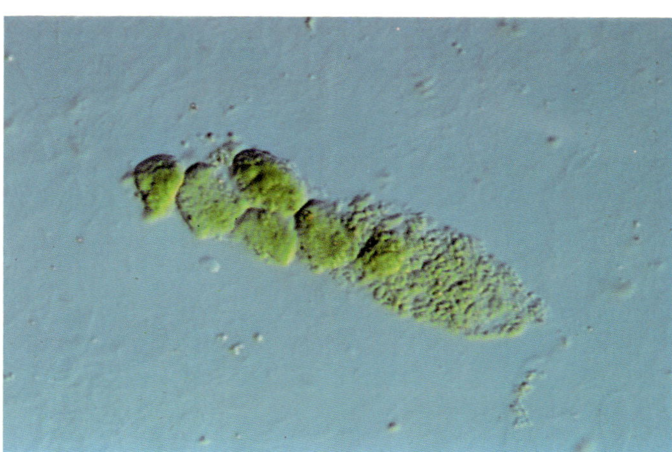

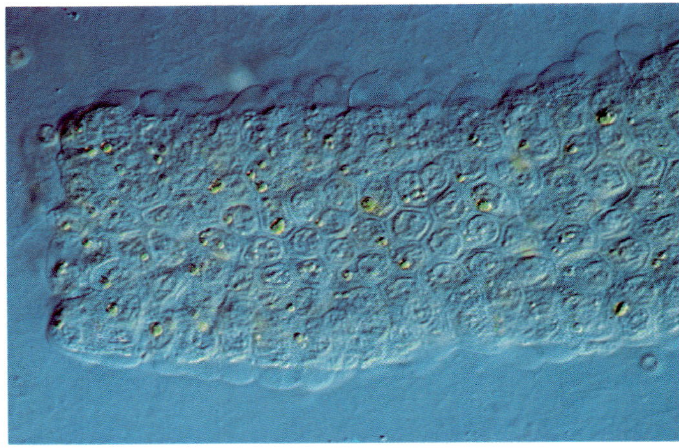

Fig 6–51. Epithelial cast, found in case of cytomegalic inclusion disease. In many well-defined epithelial cells, pale yellow irregular inclusion bodies are readily seen. Casts as well preserved as this one are not common. Each cell is prominent, as is its nucleus (ICM ×160).

Bacterial Casts

Bacterial casts appear in the urine only in pyelonephritis.[37] Bacteria have been recognized as a component part of leukocyte casts for a number of years, but their clinical significance seems to have been unappreciated by many observers. Our studies have shown that these casts are essentially pathognomonic for intrinsic renal infections and have not been observed in other forms of renal disease. Bacteria in the casts themselves may be recognized in a variety of ways but most easily by differential staining of the sediment (Figs 6–52 and 6–53).[57] These bacteria are also

Fig 6–52. Bacterial cast. Some PMNs are present in the cast, and one is adjacent to it. Close inspection shows bacillary forms scattered throughout hyaline matrix (Sternheimer-Malbin stain ×160).

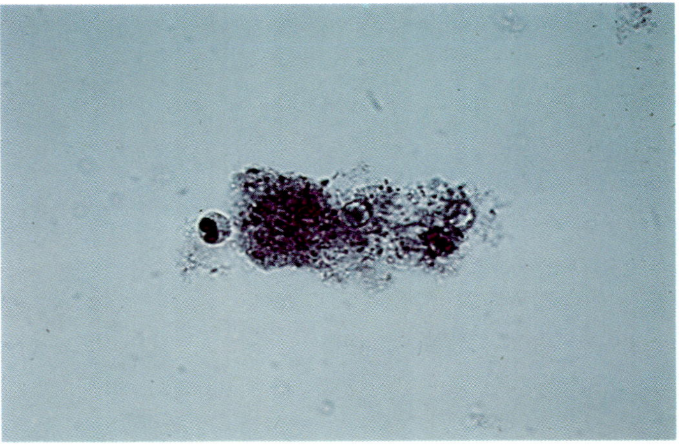

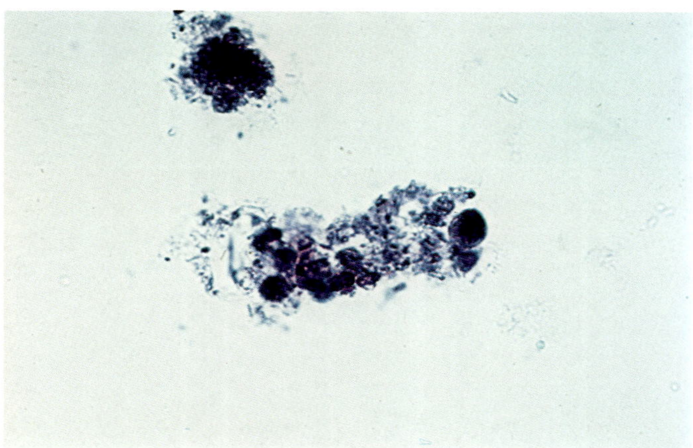

Fig 6–53. White blood cell-bacterial cast, similar to that seen in Figure 6–52. Bacteria are readily identified in the matrix, intermixed with numerous PMNs. If this cast were unstained, it would have been identified as a white cell cast, since the bacteria would appear as granules by ordinary light microscopic techniques (Sternheimer-Malbin stain ×160).

seen when either phase- or interference-contrast microscopy is used as a means of diagnosis (Fig 6–54). Unfortunately, even with the knowledge that bacteria are present in a given cast, ordinary bright-field microscopy does not permit the observer to recognize these microorganisms. Studies using SEM, which will be discussed in Chapter 7, have helped define this specific cast type.

Bacteria have been seen in casts in a pure form or accompanied by leukocytes (Fig 6–55). Many of the bacteria appear coated with a thin filamentous proteinaceous material, which seems to bind the microorganisms to the cast surface.[61] It is conceivable that this material is of renal origin and may actually be manufactured by the kidney as a type of defensive mechanism in an attempt to combat the renal infection by coating the organisms so that they may be eliminated from the body with greater facility.

Bacterial casts may be either elongate or broad, depending on the degree of renal damage. In untreated patients with pyelonephritis, these casts are almost invariably seen if the urine is carefully examined. That is not to say that all leukocyte casts in pyelonephritis patients contain bacteria. In our experience, only about one quarter of all leukocyte casts in these patients contain bacteria. After treatment with appropriate antibiotic agents, the number of bacterial casts in the sediment drops significantly, and the number of bacteria in leukocyte casts also diminishes.

Pure bacterial casts are of great interest, since often they are unrecognized and are commonly misdiagnosed as granular casts (see Fig 6–55). It is only with use of appropriate microscopic procedures or stains that the observer is able to identify them correctly. The bacteria in such a pure cast are usually closely packed together on the cast surface. However, they may be present in sparse concentrations.

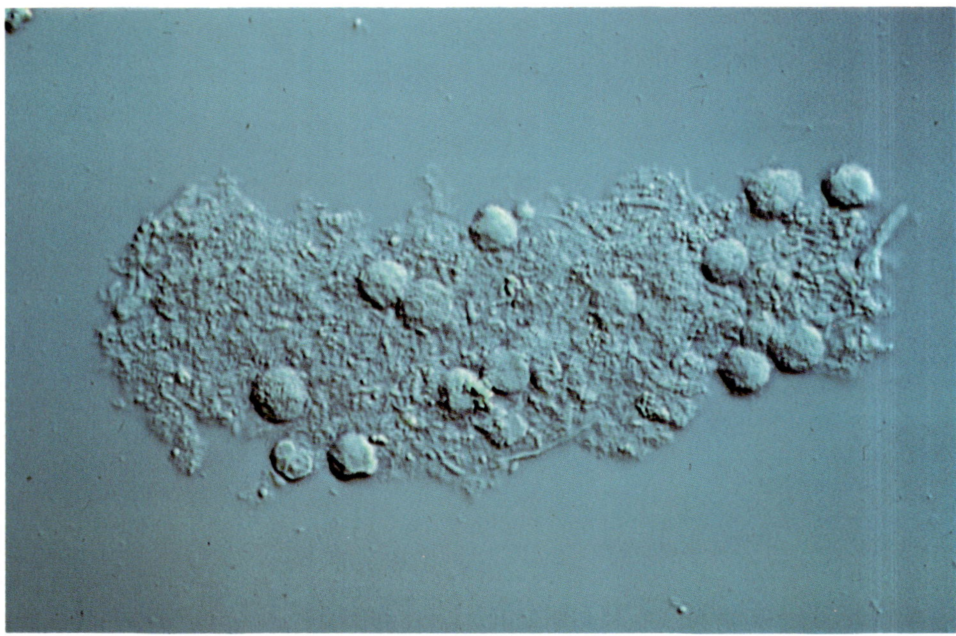

Fig 6–54. White blood cell-bacterial cast, closely correlated with an intrarenal infection. Bacillary forms are readily seen. Some leukocytes show multilobate nuclei and granular cytoplasm (ICM ×160).

Fig 6–55. Pure bacterial cast with bacillary forms easily identified throughout the cast structure (ICM ×160).

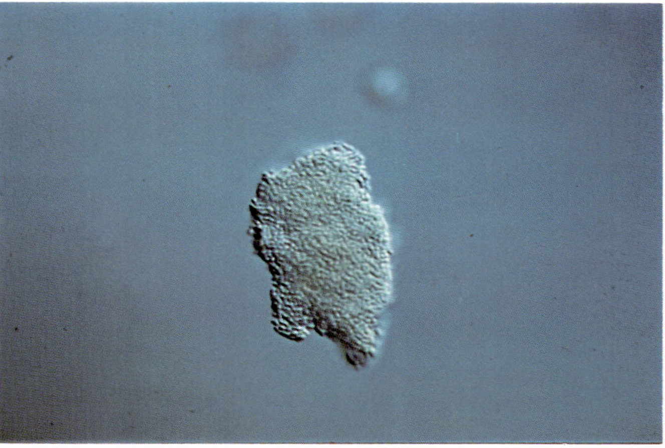

Microcrystallization or the "Crystalline Cast"

There is no such thing as a crystalline cast. The physical phenomenon of microcrystallization may occur on a preformed cast surface. This phenomenon has only recently been recognized and is not of major clinical importance. Depending on the pH of the urine, and on whether or not opportunity arises for crystals to precipitate (usually this is due to lowering of the urine temperature through refrigeration prior to analysis), certain crystals will adhere to a preexistent hyaline cast matrix and appear to be component parts of the cast itself. They are usually closely packed on the cast surface and are mostly urates, phosphates, or oxalates. They may be falsely called "pseudocasts."[28] In such instances the observer may not be able to discern whether or not a cast matrix exists beneath the external layer of crystals.

Pseudocasts are nothing more than collections of crystals (usually amorphous urates or phosphates) that have collected in a configuration simulating the appearance of a cast. For some inexplicable reason, these crystalline materials approximate themselves, one to another, to appear as cylindric, castlike objects that are easily recognized by staining (Fig 6–56). These may be easily diagnosed by using polarizing prisms, which confirm the birefringent crystalline characteristics.

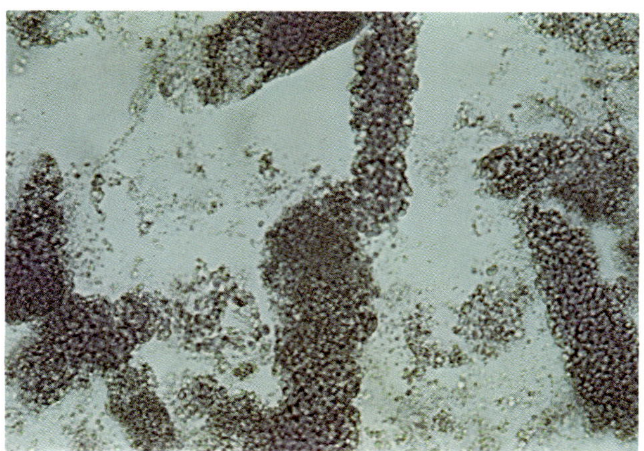

Fig 6–56. Pseudocasts, which may be easily differentiated from true casts by polarizing the urine. These crystals are birefringent, whereas true casts are not (Sternheimer-Malbin stain × 160).

7. ULTRASTRUCTURAL AND CHEMICAL STUDIES OF URINARY CASTS

Luther E. Lindner, MD, PhD

The diagnostic importance of urinary casts has long been recognized, but over the years there has been relatively little interest in more precisely defining their composition and the mechanisms by which they form. The general attitude has been that they are simply a gel of protein that molds in the lumen of the renal tubule when enough protein is present and conditions are favorable for gel formation, and that the various additional elements present are just trapped in that gel. Other varieties of casts may then form by further degenerative changes. Only recently have studies demonstrated that the composition of casts and their mode of formation are more complex. More importantly, these studies are also producing new information and insights that may have considerable diagnostic importance.

Both ultrastructural and chemical studies have contributed to this new knowledge about urinary casts. At this point ultrastructural studies have gone into greater depth, particularly those using scanning electron microscopy (SEM). Curiously, although it has been a commonly used tool for over two decades, transmission electron microscopy (TEM) has contributed very little to the understanding of casts. There has been no attempt to study casts intensively by TEM, and although casts are seen frequently in the renal tubules in biopsy specimens, to our knowledge no one has ever really attempted to observe them closely. Chemical studies have attempted to probe to greater depths, but have been seriously hampered by the inherent difficulties in directly analyzing anything as small as a cast, so they have relied in part on indirect methods such as immunofluorescence. Recent applications of the scanning electron microscope have yielded the most immediately useful information.

THE CAST MATRIX

Scanning electron micrographs have shown that the matrix of casts differs considerably from most previous concepts. The micrographs have been particularly useful here because they have produced the fundamental concept that, with only a few possible exceptions (myeloma casts and RBC casts), all casts appear to form in about the same way and appear to have the same basic matrix structure.[22] Hyaline casts will be discussed as the prototype.

Observation of a variety of hyaline casts from both normal subjects and patients shows a wide range of appearances from almost perfectly smooth surfaces to surfaces consisting of a meshwork of fibers (Fig 7–1). At first glance it is difficult to explain this range of appearances, but careful inspection shows a continuum between these two extremes, with most casts demonstrating a fibrillar structure, at least in part (Fig 7–2). Similar fibrillar protein that does not form defined structures is present in the background of the specimens. Indeed, fibrillar material is seen in the background of *all* urine specimens that contain casts.[36] Careful examination of this background protein, as well as the casts, demonstrates that the fibrils are generally smaller in diameter than the limit of resolution of the SEM used (about 10 nm) and that they are viewed as discernible fibers when they have aggregated. This being the case, the hyaline casts that appear to have perfectly smooth surfaces can be explained as casts whose fibrils are so closely packed together that the fibrillar structure cannot be resolved.

The formation of casts thus appears to be a process of condensation of a fibrillar protein to form an interlacing or interconnecting network that becomes a solid structure. The localization and concentration of protein in renal tubules long enough to condense into a defined structure is explained by the fact that the fibrils are able to adhere to the surface of the tubular epithelial cells (see Section entitled "Epithelial Casts"). The varying appearance of hyaline casts may be explained as representing stages in the process of deposition and condensation of this fibrillar matrix. Other casts form in the same way, but additional elements are incorporated into the cast.

Fig 7–1. Hyaline-epithelial cast, presumably in its early formative stages. Note matrix fibrillar material, some extending into the background, but most clearly part of the cast. A tubular epithelial cell with microvillous surface is attached to the cast by delicate fibrils (×1,000).

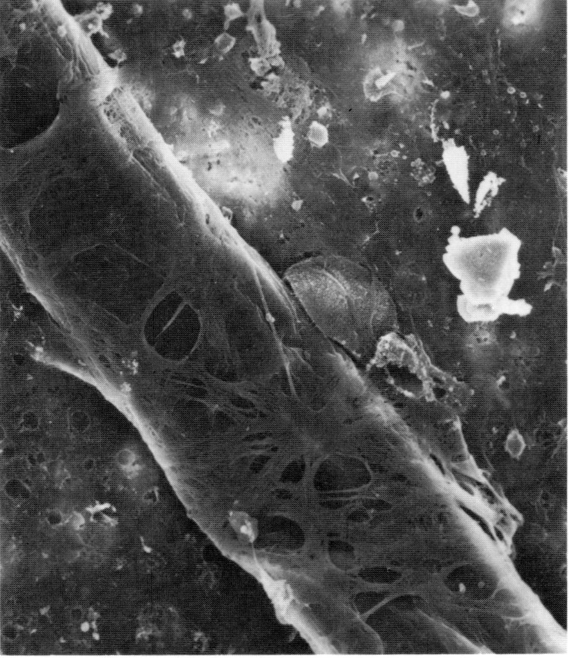

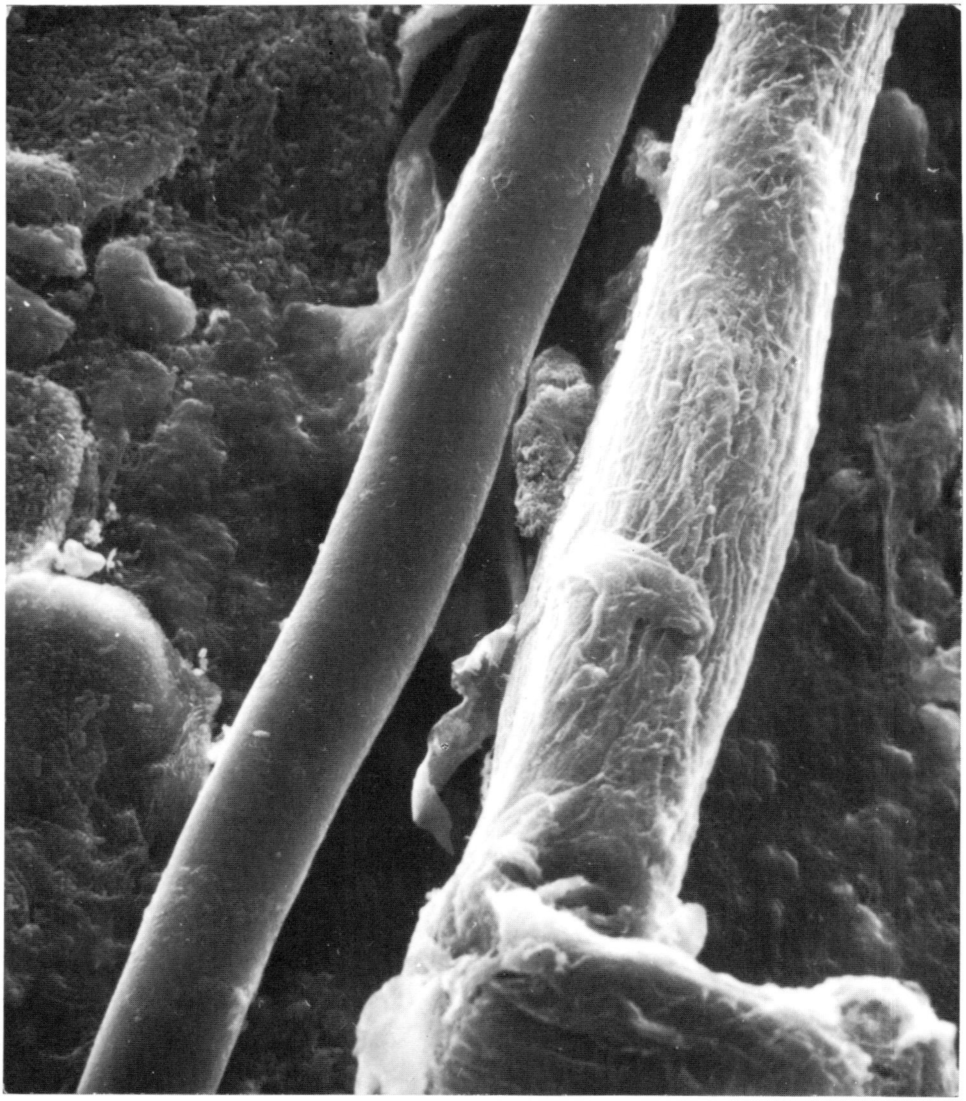

Fig 7–2. Two hyaline casts. One has a perfectly smooth surface; the other a wrinkled surface. Fibrillar structure can be recognized only in the wrinkled cast (× 1,500).

The fibrillar protein that forms the cast matrix has not been completely identified and characterized. There have been several studies using direct chemical analyses of casts or immunofluorescence.[15, 50] Both of these methods have implied that serum proteins are not ordinarily the major component of casts. These studies have demonstrated that the major component is Tamm-Horsfall protein, a fairly well characterized protein secreted by the renal tubular epithelium.[15, 41, 42, 50, 60] Although there is some debate as to exactly which portions of the nephron produce this protein, it appears that it is primarily manufactured by the epithelium lining the distal tubule and collecting ducts, and is secreted directly into the tubular lumen as a nonfibrillar monomer.[6, 43]

Tamm-Horsfall protein has some peculiar physical properties that seem largely to explain the process of cast formation as well as the labile nature of casts. The striking feature of this protein is that it reversibly aggregates into fibrillar polymers.[5, 43] Aggregation occurs under conditions of ionic strength and pH that should readily be achieved in the tubular lumen. Indeed, the aggregation occurs with such facility that it is surprising that cast formation does not occur frequently under normal conditions and produce problems by obstructing the renal tubules. Tamm-Horsfall protein is constantly being produced and excreted with only moderate variations in its level, depending on whether or not the person has been under stress or is physically ill. At any rate, aggregation of this particular protein into fibrils under appropriate conditions readily explains the process of cast formation.[43]

There are some loopholes remaining, however, in our understanding of cast formation. First, it is not clear what the specific changes are in the tubular lumen that result in the formation of a cast. Cast formation does not seem to correlate well with either pH or ionic strength (urine specific gravity or osmolarity). Studies of cast formation in persons who are under stress but otherwise healthy have shown little change in these parameters, while there is striking change in the numbers of casts produced.[23] There probably are factors involved in the process that are not understood. Another problem is that it is not at all clear whether or not Tamm-Horsfall protein is the only protein that plays a major role in cast matrix formation. Chemical studies have been largely confined to hyaline casts, so the possibility of other fibrillar proteins being involved in the formation of other types of casts is not ruled out. Immunofluorescence experiments have had limited significance in solving this issue, first because these studies have largely dealt with hyaline casts, and second because one cannot demonstrate a specific protein by immunofluorescence unless it is suspected that it is present and an appropriate antibody has been prepared. Transmission electron microscopic studies of background fibrillar urinary proteins have complicated matters by demonstrating that at least three different fibrillar urinary proteins can be recognized.[65] Even where Tamm-Horsfall is the major component of a cast, other materials might be involved, for example, by cross-linking fibrils. Clearly much work remains to be done in this area.

HYALINE CASTS

Particular notice should be taken of the ultrastructure of the hyaline cast. It is the most common type of cast present in the urine and the prototype for most other casts.[22] The appearance of hyaline casts is identical in the normal subject and the diseased patient. Both show a wide range of surfaces (Fig 7–3). It has been particularly instructive to view the casts obtained from healthy persons at timed intervals after an acute stress sufficient to stimulate them to produce urinary casts, particularly hyaline casts. Only in the early specimens may one see a high percentage of casts with a loose fibrillar structure (see Fig 7–1). After a few hours, the majority of casts have a relatively smooth surface. As time goes on, an increasing percentage of casts shows surface wrinkling. This is consistent with the theory that

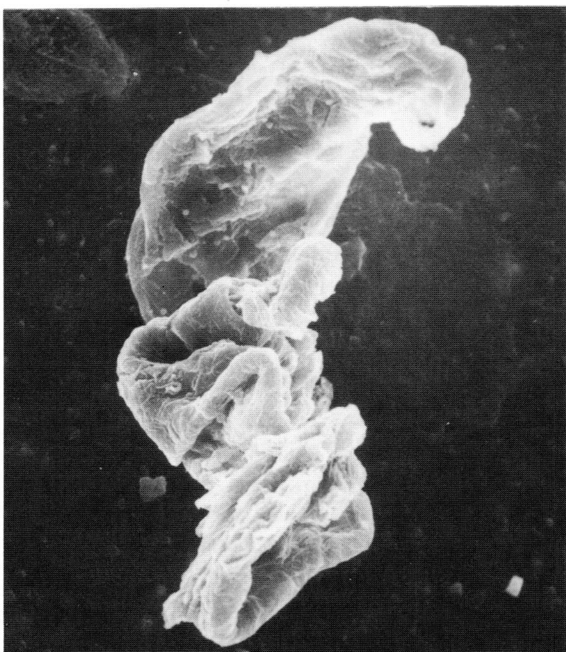

Fig 7–3. Completely wrinkled, convoluted hyaline cast. This is the least frequently seen type and presumably represents a late alteration of the cast (×1,000).

these casts are formed by precipitation and aggregation of increasing amounts of fibrillar protein until a relatively homogeneous structure is formed, and that the casts subsequently may undergo condensation and dehydration to produce wrinkling and convolution.

EPITHELIAL CASTS

Although relatively few epithelial casts have been examined ultrastructurally, those that have been studied uniformly consist of a typical hyaline cast matrix with renal tubular epithelial cells attached to the surface by delicate proteinaceous fibrils, which are sometimes very clearly demonstrated.[22] Epithelial casts have been seen only in association with disease states.

RED CELL CASTS

These consist of erythrocytes enmeshed in a fibrillar cast matrix (Fig 7–4). The cells are not merely trapped in the matrix. The matrix protein actually binds to the surface of the cells and thereby holds them tightly onto the cast as an integral part of its structure. There is a problem with the matrix of the red cell cast. It cannot

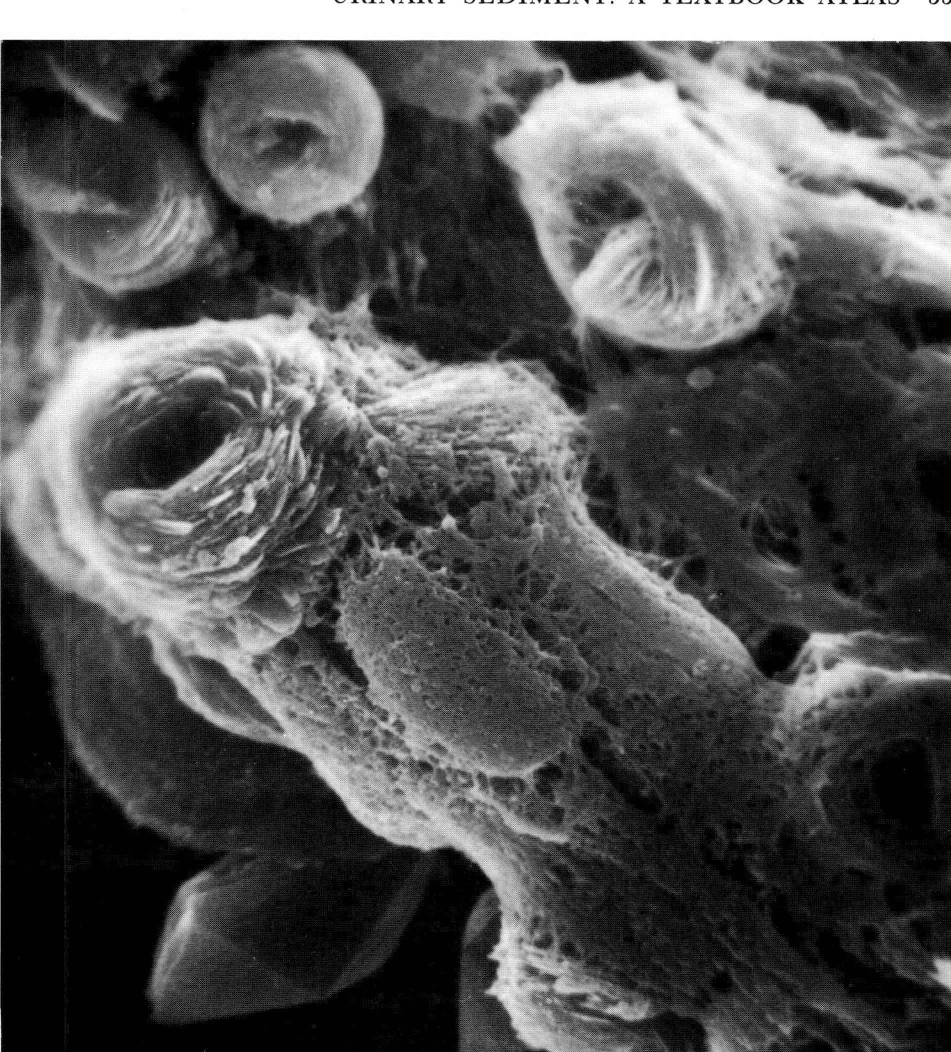

Fig 7–4. Red cell cast. Red cells are tightly enmeshed in fibrillar matrix, which is tightly attached to their surface. A calcium oxalate crystal is seen in the background (×5,000).

be distinguished by SEM from the matrix of other casts, but, in general, red cells cannot enter the tubule lumen unless there is a defect or a break in a glomerular or tubular basement membrane. With such a break, all serum proteins, including fibrinogen, would also be expected to enter the lumen. It is therefore likely that the matrix of RBC casts contains at least some fibrin.

WHITE CELL CASTS

White cell casts also consist of cells enmeshed in a fibrillar matrix (Fig 7–5). They differ from red cell casts in several ways. The leukocytes are usually less tightly bound in the cast structure and may have some surface areas free of attached fibrils. The cast matrix itself is usually much looser and less well formed than in the RBC cast. The leukocytes may be granulocytes or lymphocytes, or a mixture of the two. Macrophages are rarely seen. The granulocytes often show all stages of degeneration, with holes in the plasma membrane, loss of plasma membrane, and release of granules. The looseness of the matrix in many white cell casts may be the result of the release of hydrolytic enzymes from the leukocytes.

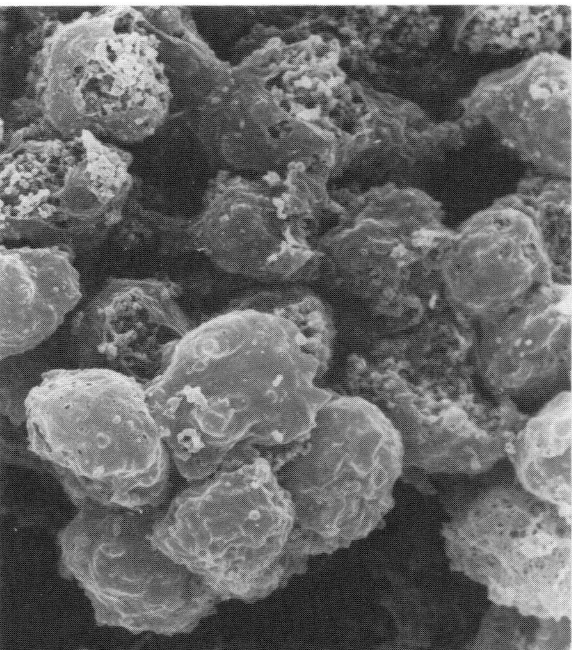

Fig 7–5. White cell cast. White cells are held in fibrillar matrix. They do not have as much surface material as red cell casts, but fibrillar matrix is also attached to their surface. Varying degrees of cell degeneration are seen with pits, holes, and large membranous ruptures (×2,500).

GRANULAR CASTS

Granular casts have traditionally been thought to arise from the degeneration of cellular casts. Recent studies have cast doubt on this theory, at least in part. There is clearly more than one type of granular cast, and they probably arise in more than one way.

Some granular casts appear to consist of a typical hyaline cast matrix to which a relatively uniform-appearing granule has been added (Fig 7–6). The number of

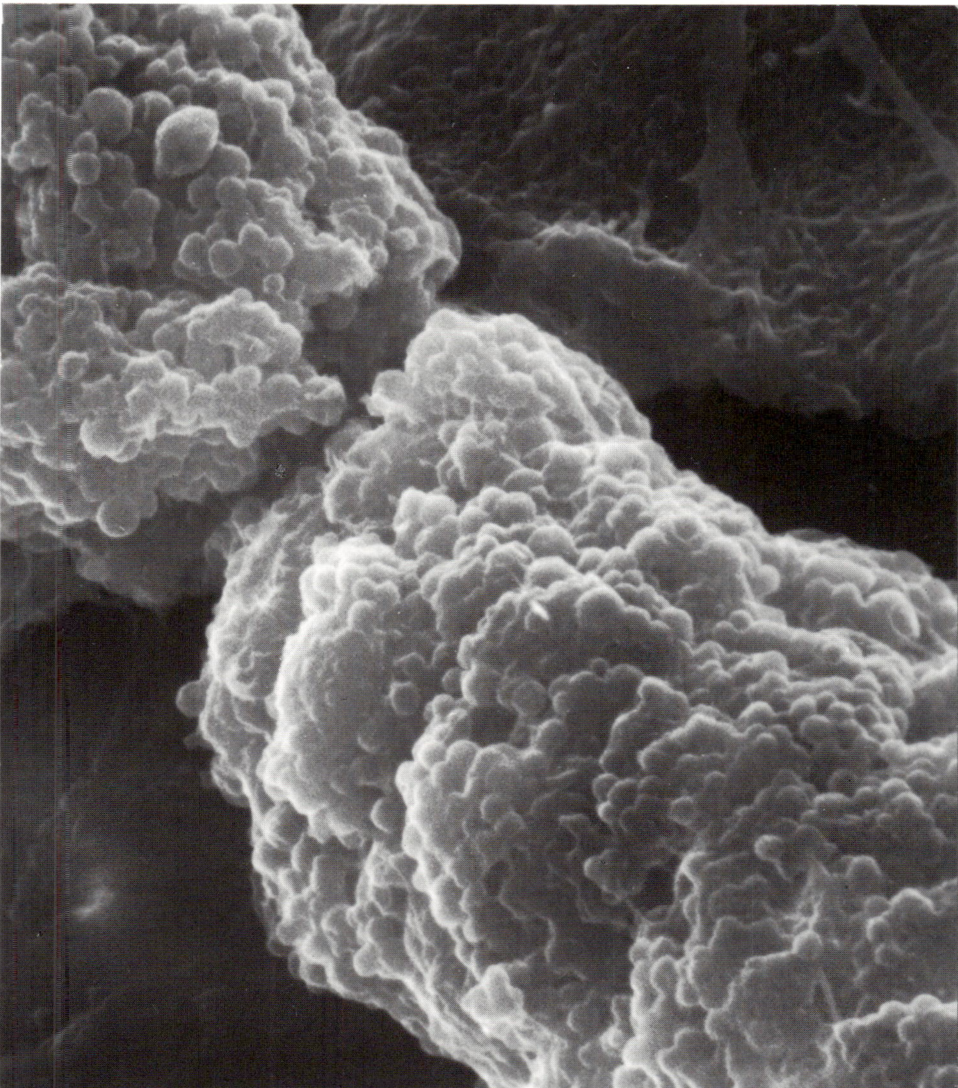

Fig 7–6. Granular cast with relatively uniform granules embedded in the matrix. The cast is fractured, demonstrating that the granules extend throughout the interior. A squamous cell is in the background (×6,500).

these granules is quite variable. This type of cast is present in both normal subjects and patients. The exact chemical nature of these granules is unknown, although it has been speculated that they may be products of the renal tubular epithelium. Immunofluorescence has shown that serum proteins may be a major component. Another commonly identified granular cast appears to arise from the degeneration of cellular (especially granulocyte-containing) casts (Fig 7–7). These are seen only in disease states.

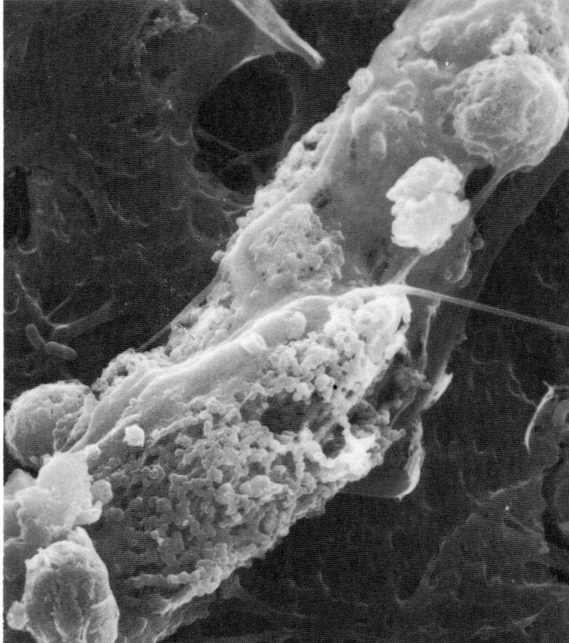

Fig 7–7. White cell-granular cast. In addition to the same features seen in Figure 7–5, there are localized granular collections that appear to stem from white cell breakdown (×3,000).

A type of cast that has been mistaken by light microscopy for a granular cast is the bacterial cast. Here, SEM studies have aptly demonstrated the bacterial component.[37] There may still be other types of granular casts that have not yet been distinguished.

WAXY CASTS

Waxy casts have traditionally been thought to arise by the degeneration of cellular casts, but SEM studies make it very clear that this is usually not the case.[22] Waxy casts have a fibrillar matrix; to this a material has been added which, at the limit of resolution of the SEM, is completely featureless and waxy (Fig 7–8). The material is frequently deposited in plates and appears to be present particularly on the cast surface. At this time the nature and source of this material are unknown. Waxy casts have not been observed in normal subjects.

FATTY CASTS

Fatty casts have not been studied ultrastructurally. Since the solvents ordinarily used in processing for either SEM or TEM remove any lipid from the casts, it may not be possible to study this type of cast ultrastructurally except in specially processed specimens and with any associated artifacts.

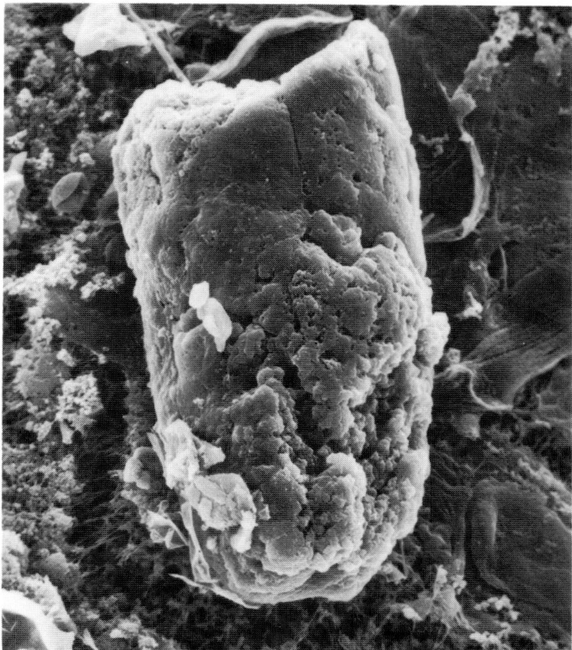

Fig 7–8. Waxy cast. Amorphous material has been added to fibrillar matrix, suggesting surface deposits. Some granules are also seen (×1,000).

BACTERIAL CASTS

Casts containing bacteria have occasionally been seen in the past by light microscopy, but they were considered rare and of little importance. It was only when SEM was applied to the sediments of patients with acute pyelonephritis that it was recognized that these casts are by no means rare but are present in the urine of most, if not all, patients with pyelonephritis.[37] Ultrastructurally, they consist of bacteria bound tightly into a fibrillar matrix by fibrils attached to and coating their surface. The fibrillar cast matrix is sometimes very loose. Two main varieties have been seen: (1) pure bacterial casts that contain no other elements, which are relatively uncommon (Fig 7–9); and (2) casts in which bacteria are admixed with granulocytes, which often show degeneration (Fig 7–10). Rarely are additional leukocytic cell types present. These casts have been seen only in pyelonephritis and appear to be specifically diagnostic of this condition. Furthermore, it has been shown that SEM is not needed for their identification. They are not readily seen by ordinary bright-field microscopy, such as is routinely used for urinalysis. Viewed in this way, these casts are not distinguishable from granular casts. But when viewed by phase-contrast or interference-contrast microscopy, or with staining of the sediment, they are readily identified, usually without prolonged searching.

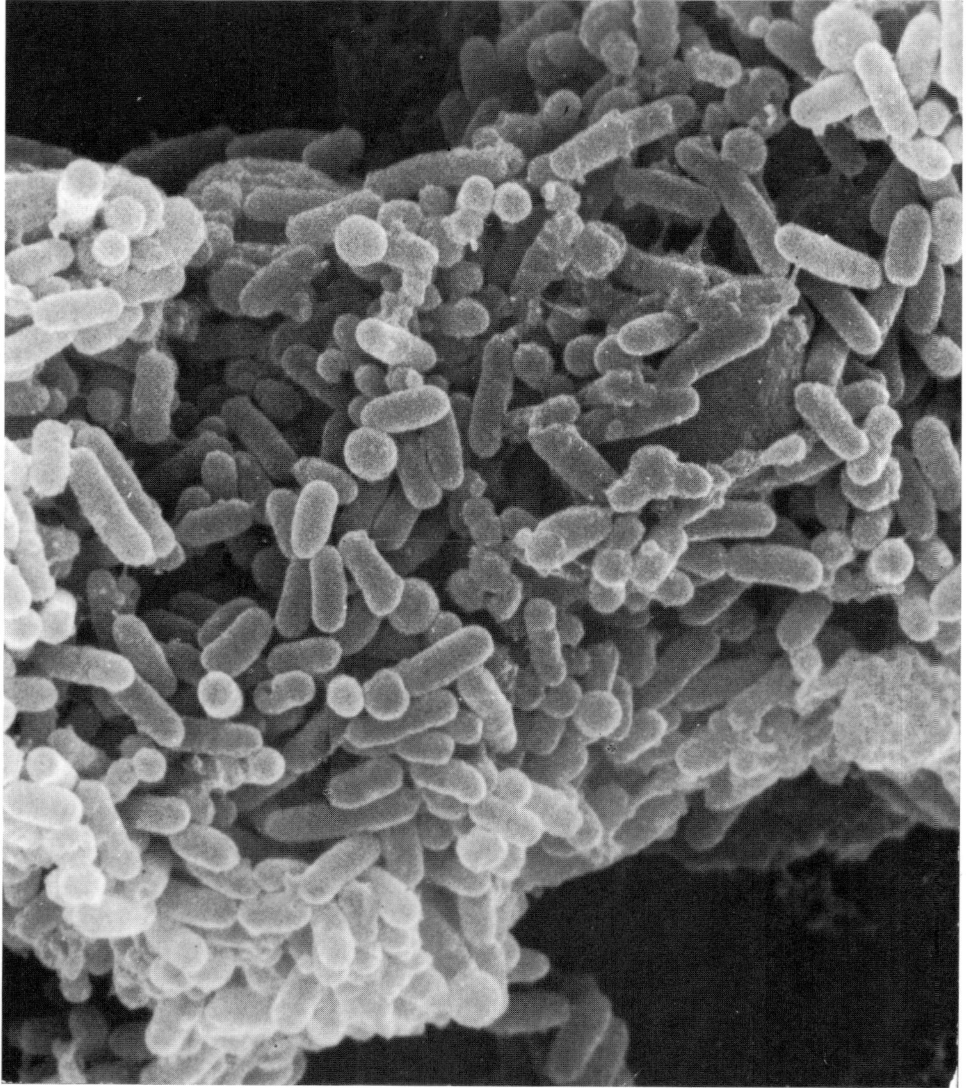

Fig 7–9. Pure bacterial cast. Bacteria are held together by fibrillar matrix, which is indiscernible here but evident in other examples (×8,200).

MIXED CASTS

As one might predict from what has been said, there is a fundamental underlying hyaline framework to all casts. Special types differ only by what is added to the matrix. Mixed types of casts can be observed to contain various cellular elements, granules, waxy material, etc, in any combination imaginable. These elements do not appear to have any special significance.

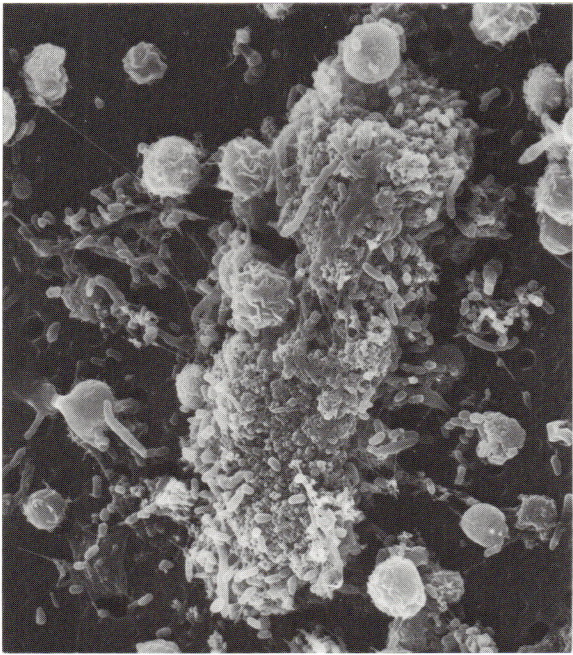

Fig 7–10. Mixed bacterial-white cell cast. More common than the pure bacterial cast, it differs from that shown in Figure 7–9 by having more matrix, which contains some cast-bound white cells (×1,500).

MYELOMA CASTS

To date, very few myeloma casts have been examined ultrastructurally, and no results have been published. Preliminary studies indicate that myeloma casts differ significantly from all other casts. They are formed from a granular-fibrillar matrix that has a distinctly different appearance from the matrix of other casts. The same matrix material is present in the background in large quantities and probably represents protein fibrils of light chains. Further study is expected to document more fully the unique nature of this material.

SUMMARY

In summary, recent studies of urinary casts, particularly those using SEM, are adding greatly to our knowledge of how casts form, of their composition, and of their diagnostic importance. Indeed, the recognition of the bacterial cast and its clinical importance represents the first instance in which examination of the urine for casts can render a specific clinical diagnosis.

8. PARASITES IN URINE

Donald C. Cannon, MD, PhD

Protozoan and metazoan parasites are rarely observed in the urine. *Trichomonas vaginalis* is the only exception to this general rule. Parasites appearing in the urinary sediment can originate from the genitourinary tract, including the accessory male reproductive organs; from the vagina; from the perineal or pubic skin or hair; or may be present because of fecal contamination.

T vaginalis primarily infests the deeper vagina and cervix, including the endocervical glands. However, this organism is readily capable of involving the urethra, periurethral glands, and urinary bladder in both sexes, and the prostate. Although mild infestations can be asymptomatic, large numbers of parasites typically cause vaginitis with associated clinical symptoms of a profuse, watery or creamy, frothy vaginal discharge; vaginal burning; vulvar irritation and itching; and dyspareunia. Both men and women may also experience a mild urethral discharge, urinary frequency, and dysuria. Organisms in the urinary sediment may therefore originate from either the urinary tract or the vagina.

Being quite common and the only flagellate found in the urine, *T vaginalis* is easily identified (Figs 8–1 and 8–2). Phase-contrast microscopy enhances the recognition of these parasites. The organisms are spheric or pear-shaped and usually

Fig 8–1. *Trichomonas vaginalis* in urine, easily identified due to its motility, flagella, and pear shape. A squamous cell is present for size comparison (BF ×250).

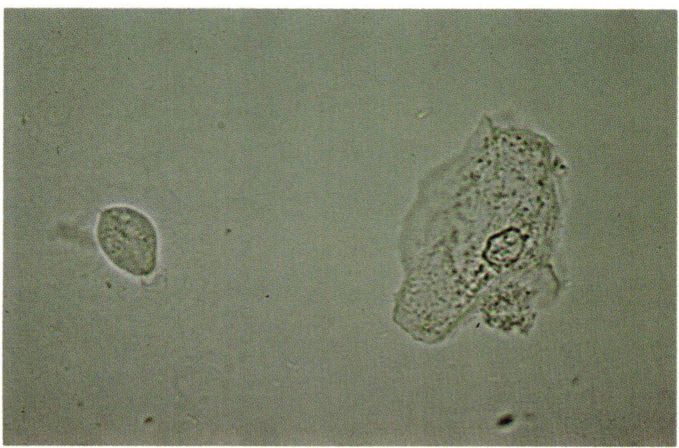

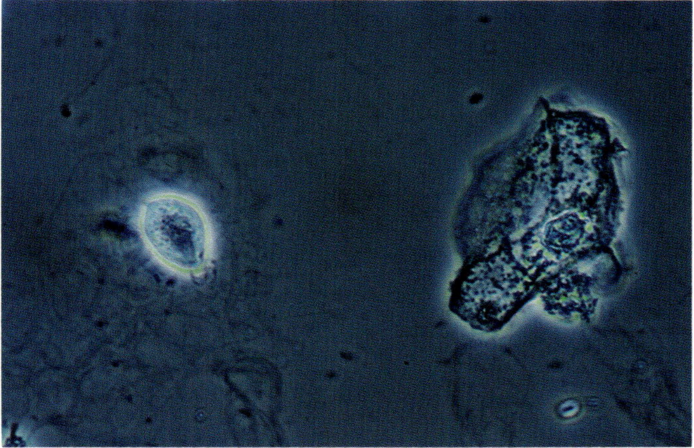

Fig 8–2. *Trichomonas vaginalis*. Flagella are readily distinguished, thereby facilitating a specific, accurate diagnosis (PH ×250).

15–20 μ long, although they may measure 10–30 μ. There are two pairs of anteriorly situated flagella and a short midline undulating membrane, which usually extends for only about one half the length of the body. Together these organelles propel the organisms forward in a rapid, jerking motion combined with a more gentle rotation. The oval nucleus is relatively indistinct because of sparse chromatin. The cytoplasm typically contains numerous granules and at least a few food vacuoles.

Trichomoniasis is usually accompanied by a marked exudation of polymorphonuclear leukocytes, which may also appear in the urine frequently with increased numbers of red blood cells. Polymorphonuclear neutrophils can exhibit cellular changes in the presence of trichomonads that are similar to those exhibited cytologically by exfoliated squamous cells—enlarged nuclei with prominent condensation of chromatin about the nuclear membrane so that the nucleus appears sharply demarcated with a hollow-looking interior.

Enterobius vermicularis, commonly called pinworm, threadworm, or seatworm, primarily infests the cecum and vermiform appendix, particularly in children (Fig 8–3). Gravid female helminths migrate to the anus, where they deposit ova on the perianal skin, especially at night. Uncommonly the worms migrate to the vulva and enter the vagina, causing clinically significant vaginitis in addition to the common symptoms of perianal pruritis, nervousness, and restlessness. It is rare for the pinworm ova or the adult worm to be detected in the urinary sediment. The ova of *E vermicularis* measure about 25 × 50 μ. Adult females are 8–13 mm long, while males are only 2–5 mm (Fig 8–4).

The parasite indigenous to the urinary tract that is of greatest importance on a worldwide basis is *Schistosoma hematobium*. This trematode cannot be transmitted in the United States because of the absence of a suitable species of snail available to serve as an intermediate host. It does infest vast numbers of persons in Africa and Southwestern Asia, particularly in Egypt, Syria, Iraq, and Iran. The adult worms live in the pelvic veins where the females deposit their ova directly into the

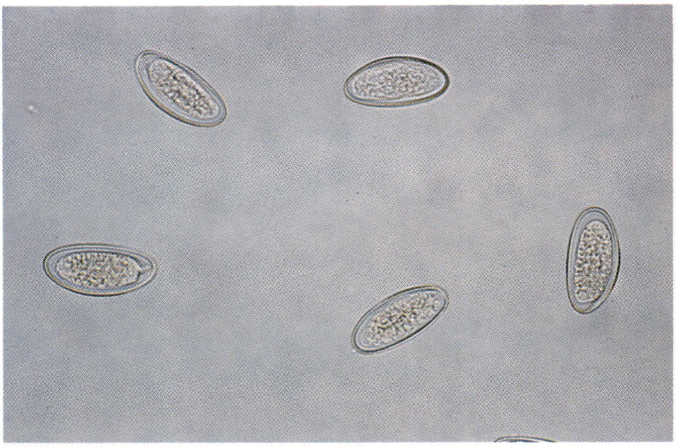

Fig 8–3. *Enterobius vermicularis* (pinworm), occasionally seen in adults but more frequently in children. Ova are elliptic with one side somewhat flatter than the other (BF ×100).

wall of the urinary bladder, ureters, or urethra. The ova eventually are discharged into the urine. Relatively few ova are deposited per unit of time, so ova tend to be scarce in the urine.

The ova of *S hematobium* are distinguished from those of *S mansoni* and *S japonicum* by the presence of a small but distinct terminal spine (Fig 8–5). The ovum is characteristically about 150 μ in length by 50 μ in cross diameter. Detection of the infestation is sometimes enhanced by adding fresh water to the urine sediment. This causes the eggs to hatch into ciliated, actively motile *miracidia,* which are barely visible to the naked eye.

Mites can occasionally be found in the urinary sediment as a result of falling into the urine from the skin of the pubic and perineal areas during collection. Various species attack humans, but the most common is *Sarcoptes scabei,* which causes

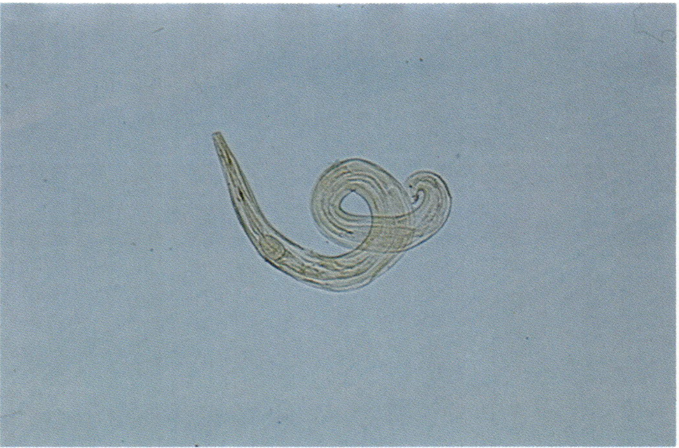

Fig 8–4. *Enterobius vermicularis,* adult male. Smaller than its female adult counterpart, it measures 2–5 mm (BF ×13).

Fig 8–5. *Schistosoma haematobium* ovum. Note small but distinct terminal spine (BF ×40).

scabies or "the itch." Adult female mites burrow into the skin about the body, including the external genitalia of both men and women, to deposit their ova. The ova hatch into larvae, which resemble adult mites except for the absence of a well developed fourth pair of legs. Either larvae or adults appear in the urine. Adult males measure about 0.25 mm in length, and the adult females about 0.3–0.4 mm (Fig 8–6).

Another arthropod parasite that can be found as a "drop-in" in the urine sediment is the crab louse, *Phthirus pubis,* which preferentially lives in pubic hair. Crab lice are readily distinguished from mites by their greater size (Fig 8–7). The adult females, which are somewhat larger than males, are about 1.5–2.0 mm long.

Various other protozoa and helminth ova can occasionally be found in the urine sediment when fecal contamination of the urine occurs in infested persons.

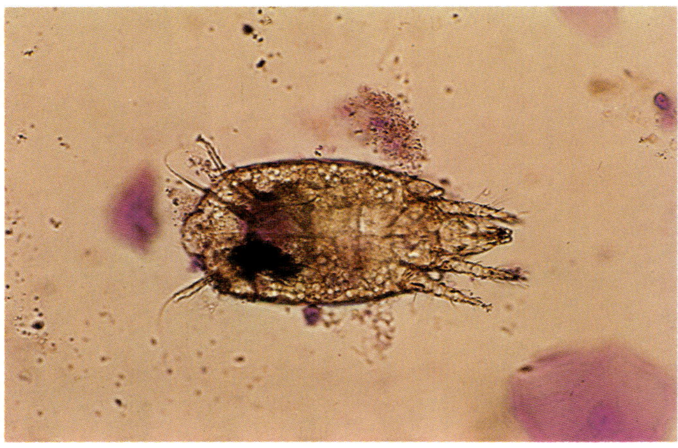

Fig 8–6. Adult mite, which is rarely found in the urinary sediment (Sternheimer-Malbin stain ×100).

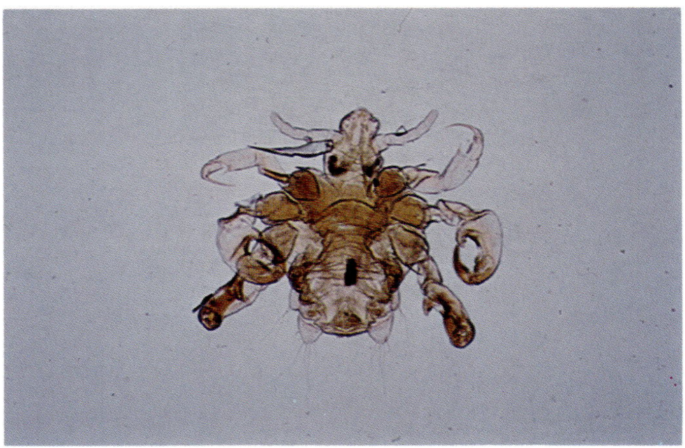

Fig 8–7. *Pediculosis pubis* (pubic louse), a rare contaminant in urine because it usually drops from the pubic hair during collection (BF ×100).

9. ARTIFACTS AND EXOGENOUS ELEMENTS OF THE URINARY SEDIMENT

Donald C. Cannon, MD, PhD

Various materials and substances can occur in the urinary sediment that are not endogenous to the urinary tract per se. These may be from the male reproductive organs, the vagina or vulva, the skin, the feces, or the environment.

Residual spermatozoa are flushed from the male urethra by the urine stream following ejaculation. Spermatozoa from the vagina are frequently found in the urine of females following coitus. Similarly, microcalculi, the "corpora amylacea" of the prostate, may be washed from the male urethra subsequent to ejaculation.[53] These calculi range greatly in size and may measure up to several hundred microns in diameter. Typically, prostatic concretions have indistinct concentric laminations (Fig 9–1). They are infrequently present in the urine and have little pathologic significance.

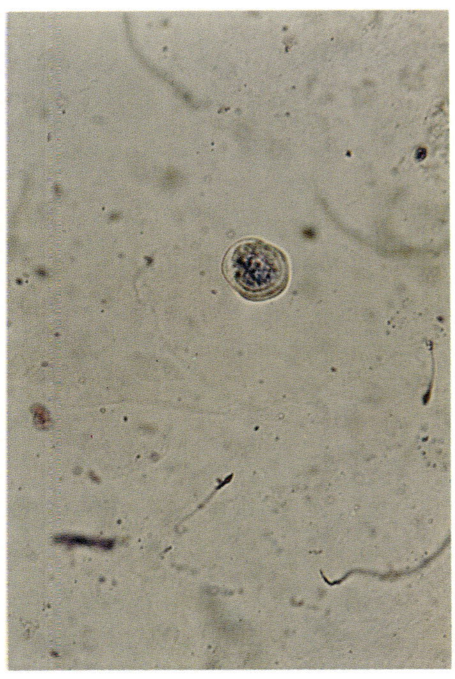

Fig 9–1. Corpora amylacea from the prostate, reflecting urine contamination with semen (BF ×160).

Fecal material can usually be identified by its brown coloration, the assortment of bizarre shapes and sizes of component elements, and large cuboidal to columnar cells, including goblet cells (Fig 9–2). Fecal contamination of urine most often occurs in incontinent babies or elderly persons. More infrequently, a fistulous communication between the urinary tract and the intestines exists.

Talcum powder, commonly used as a dusting powder to prevent chafing or heat rash, appears in the urine sediment as colorless to pale brown, amorphous crystals (Fig 9–3). Because talc consists primarily of magnesium silicate, it readily polarizes light.

An absorbable combination of amylose and amylopectin derived from cornstarch is used as a dusting powder for surgical gloves. Not infrequently it enters the urine container during catheterization. The starch granules are usually identifiable by their size, shape, and high refractive index (Fig 9–4). Definitive identification is achieved by staining the granules dark brown to black with iodine solution and noting birefringence with polarized light (Figs 9–5 and 9–6).

Diatoms and pollen can enter urine containers from either clothing or skin. Diatoms are unicellular algae that are normally found in both fresh and salt water. They vary greatly in size and have delicate but distinct cell walls of silica. Most species are much larger than human cells and may measure up to 80 μ in length

Fig 9–2 ***(left).*** Fecal contamination of urine. The totally bizarre nature of this sediment and brownish color facilitate the diagnosis (BF ×40).

Fig 9–3 ***(right).*** Talc granules in urine. Some leukocytes are also present (BF ×128).

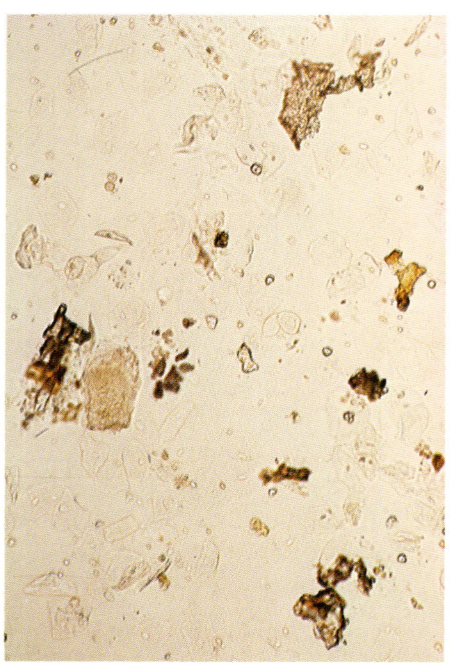

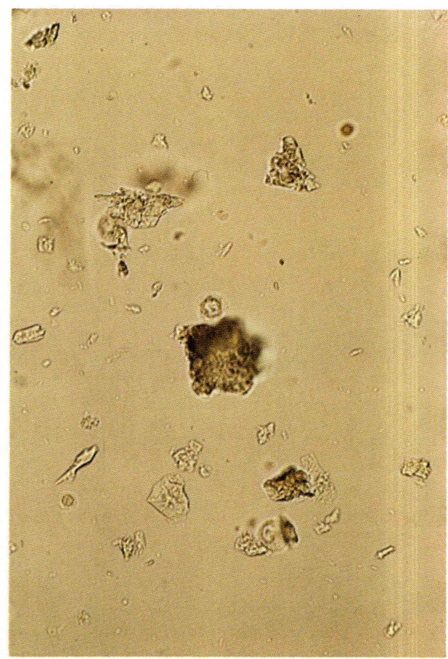

(Fig 9–7). Plant cells, including pollen grains, also have a wide range of sizes, although their large size differentiates them from human cells. They are further recognized as nonhuman by their distinct cell walls—often double layered—and central, large nucleus (Figs 9–8 and 9–9). They are infrequently found in urine as contaminants.

On the other hand, hair and cotton fibers frequently appear in the urine sediment. Ordinarily, plant and animal fibers are easily recognized and not confused with casts. They have a high refractive index, may have anisotropic properties, and are usually of great length when compared with urinary casts (Figs 9–10 and 9–11).

One interesting artifact that can prove very puzzling is created by precipitation of Sternheimer-Malbin stain. Crystal lattices in the form of needles or complexes resembling sea urchins occur. These should not be mistaken for abnormal urinary crystals. Often, various stains, especially those used in the preparation of urinary sediments, will crystallize and simulate the appearance of certain pathologic structures such as various abnormal crystals (Fig 9–12). The observer must be extremely careful not to misdiagnose such crystalline artifacts as abnormal crystals.

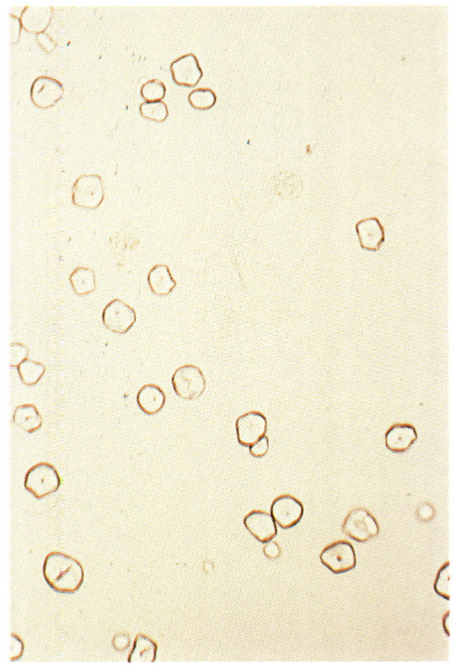

Fig 9–4. Starch granules, relatively regular spherules derived from cornstarch and commonly found in urine (BF ×100).

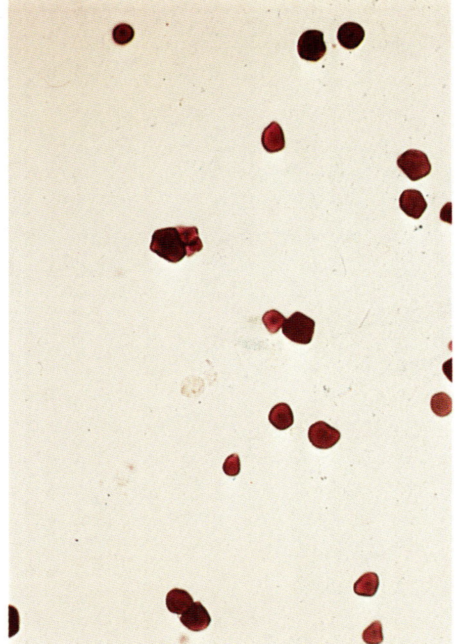

Fig 9–5. Starch granules in urine stained with iodine (BF $\times 100$).

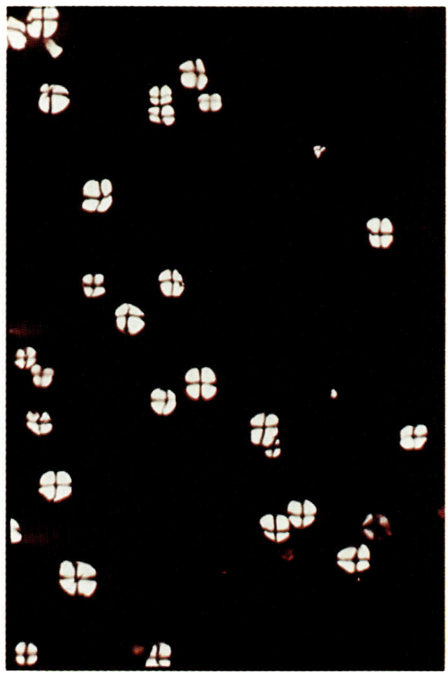

Fig 9–6. Starch granules in urine, polarized. Care must be taken not to misidentify these granules as oval fat bodies or free urinary lipid granules. Birefringent pattern is different with urinary lipids (Pol $\times 100$).

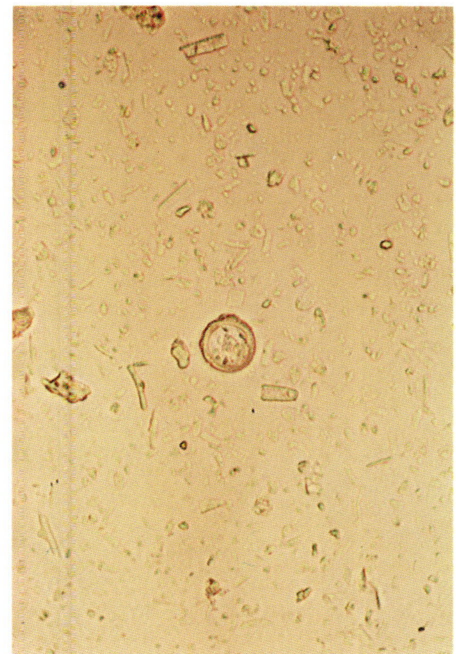

Fig 9–7. Diatom, a rare contaminant in urine (BF ×205).

Fig 9–8. Plant cell and white blood cells with numerous PMNs in urine (BF ×200).

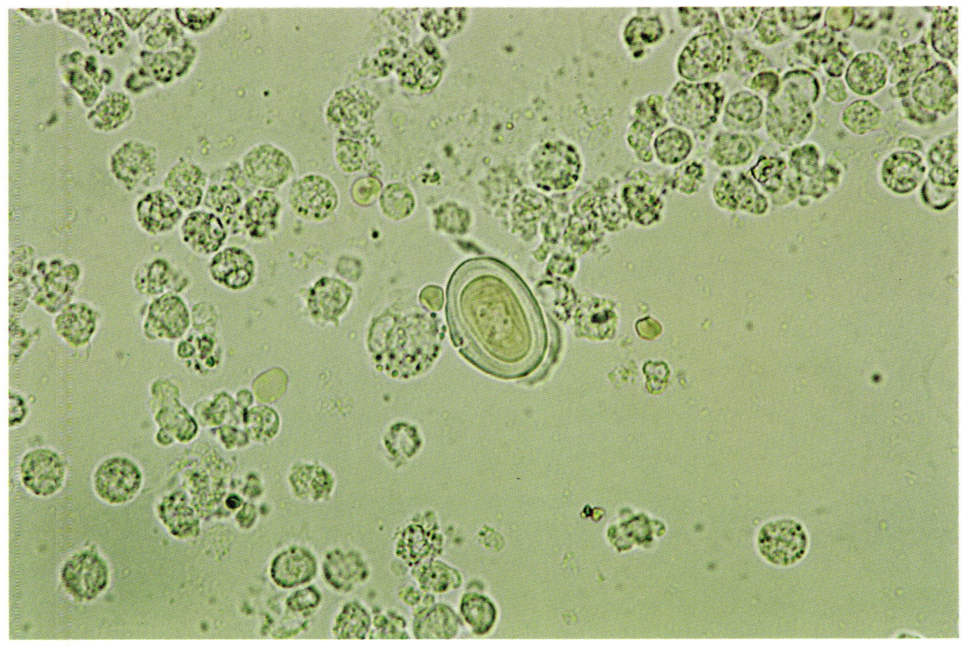

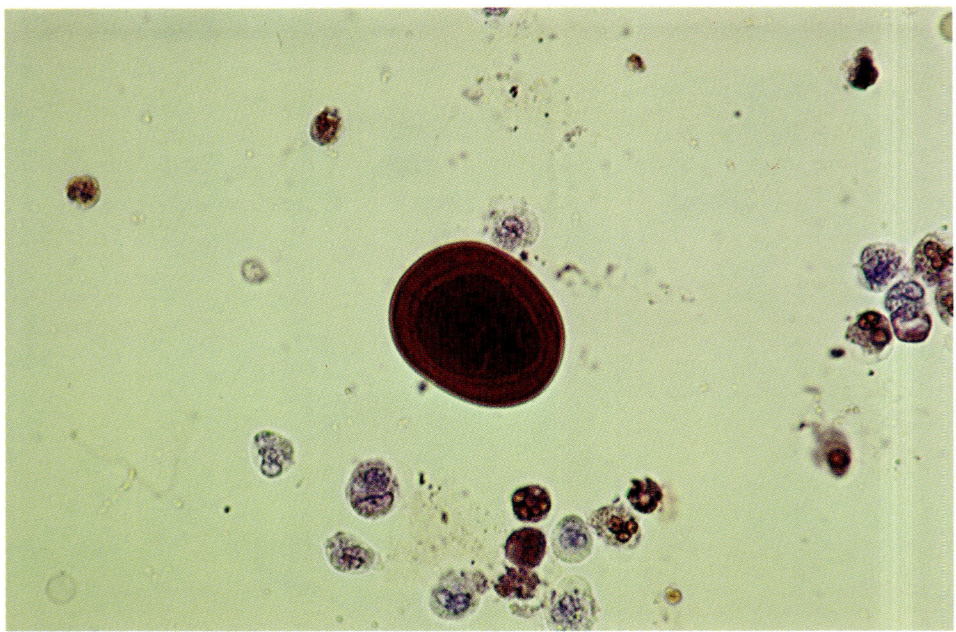

Fig 9–9. Plant cell and white blood cells in urine. The plant cell (center) is easily distinguished from a human cell by its great size, massive nucleus, and thick walls (Sternheimer-Malbin stain ×250).

Fig 9–10. Cotton fiber (BF ×51).

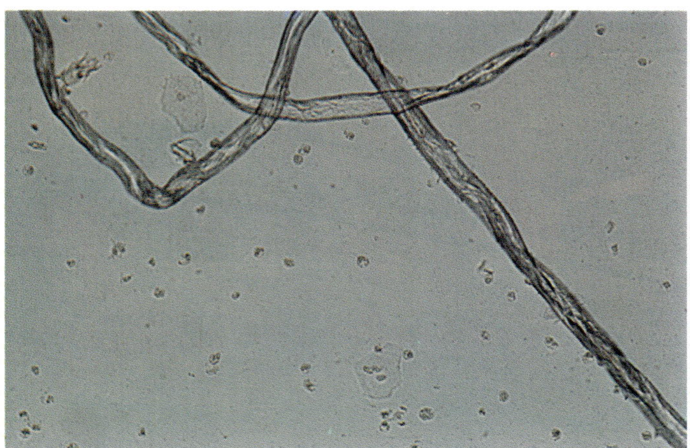

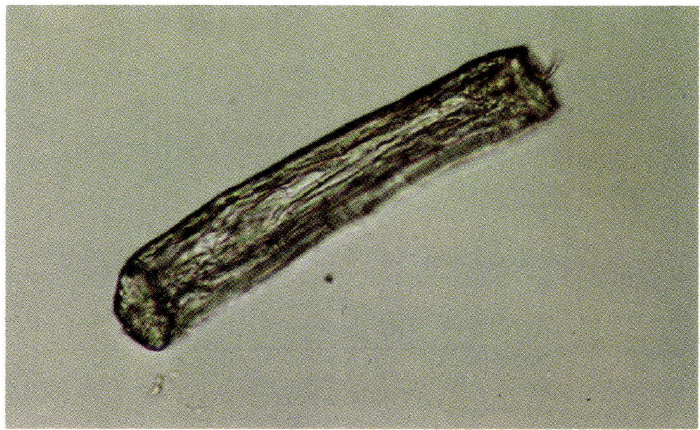

Fig 9–11. Fiber artifact, closely simulating a urinary cast. However, its high refractive index, birefringence in polarized light, and brittleness distinguish it from a pathologic entity (BF ×200).

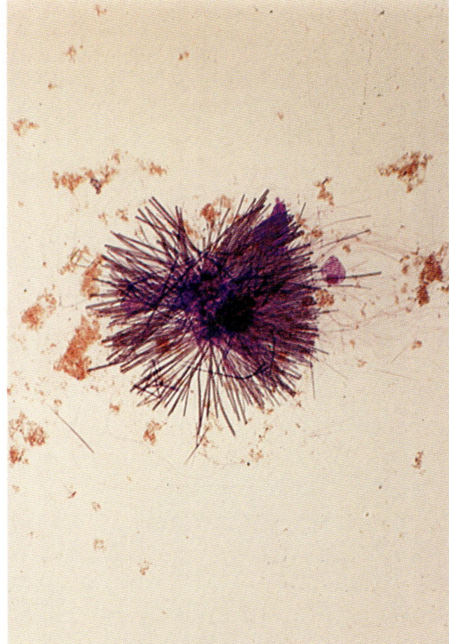

Fig 9–12. Crystalline artifact in urine (Sternheimer-Malbin stain ×100).

10. QUALITY ASSURANCE IN URINALYSIS

The urinalysis section of the laboratory should be involved in a quality assurance (QAS) program so that accuracy, precision, and reproducibility of results can be assured. Although the microscopic evaluation of the urinary sediment is considered by some to be somewhat subjective, or at best semiquantitative, a comprehensive QAS program will ensure that the results obtained from sediment examination will at least be consistent on a day-to-day basis. Commercial materials are available to assist the laboratory in implementing such a program. However, laboratorians can implement it by their own efforts. Basically, a QAS program for urinalysis can be defined as *doing the same thing to every specimen under controlled conditions every day, from the time the specimen is voided until it is observed under the microscope and reported*. Standardization of each step of the urinalysis procedure is thus a necessity for accurate and reproducible results.[21]

Perhaps the most important aspect of a proper microscopic examination of the urinary sediment is that the specimen be acceptable for inspection. This implies prompt processing after voiding, submission to the laboratory expeditiously, and review by the laboratory technologist within a reasonably short period after receipt. Criteria need to be developed for rejection of specimens. A specimen that has been left at room temperature for several hours will become contaminated by microorganisms. If any proteinaceous components are present, these will inevitably be destroyed by proteolytic enzymes present in the urine, as well as by bacterial products. It is therefore incumbent on the laboratory to demand and implement proper collection techniques (clean-catch specimens wherever possible or catheterized specimens), collection of a sufficient volume of urine, rapid dispatch to the laboratory, and prompt examination. Needless to say, if the specimen is not properly labeled with the patient's name, it should be rejected.

Urine should be centrifuged prior to microscopic examination. Although this is not done routinely in all countries of the world, it is accepted practice in the United States. Centrifugation provides a concentrated specimen for the examiner to observe and offers less chance of missing important elements. To achieve quality assurance when centrifugation is used in the laboratory for microscopic sediment evaluation, a standardized and well calibrated centrifuge is essential. The same measured aliquot of urine should always be used, and the time of centrifugation should be constant. The actual volume of urine used for centrifugation is not critical. Most laboratories have adopted a volume of 10–12 ml. Centrifugation time and centrifugal force on the head should be calculated beforehand and implemented so as not to pack the elements too closely in the bottom of the centrifuge tube and to avoid their destruction by a too rapid or prolonged spin. If sufficient volume cannot be obtained from the urine specimen to meet the standards previously adopted in the laboratory, the urine should be diluted with an aliquot of saline to provide such volume in the centrifuge tube. In such circumstances—especially in pediatric patients where volumes are often less than necessary—saline should be added to the urine sample and appropriate dilution factors taken into account when the sediment elements are quantitated on reporting.

For semiquantitative sediment evaluation, a standardized volume of urine (already concentrated in the centrifuge tube) should be observed under a coverslip. Commercially available plastic slides (Kova)* with standardized-volume observation chambers may be used for this purpose. On the other hand, a similar effect is achieved by using glass pipettes of uniform bore and length, which deliver approximately 0.05 ml. When a coverslip is applied over this volume of urine, microscopic observations are consistent.

Microscopic reporting of the numbers and types of sediment elements present is of importance. Ordinarily, cells are counted as numbers per high-power microscopic field.[16, 28] The exact magnification varies with each microscope used. However, the usual high-power microscopic field includes an objective of 40 times magnification and an ocular of ten times. Again, QAS procedures dictate that the microscopic field be the same for all urine specimens; therefore, the microscope used on a day-to-day basis should not be switched.

Some comment should be made at this point about the microscope in sediment evaluation. A modern binocular microscope is mandatory. It should be provided with built-in controls that can focus the light source, alter the intensity, and provide a high degree of contrast. In addition, it is desirable to have equipment for the performance of phase-contrast, interference-contrast, and polarized microscopy. The lenses and condensers should be clean.

If these basic principles of quality assurance are followed in the urinalysis laboratory, the data obtained from any given examination can be expected to be both accurate and reproducible, and the procedure and its results will prove to be a valuable adjunct to the care of the patient.

---

*ICL Scientific, Fountain Valley, CA 92708.

REFERENCES

1. Addis T: The effect of some physiological variables on the number of casts, red blood cells, white blood cells and epithelial cells in the urine of normal individuals. J Clin Invest 2:417–421, 1926
2. Addis T: Glomerular Nephritis: Diagnosis and Treatment. New York: Macmillan Publishing Co, Inc, 1948
3. Addis T: The number of formed elements in the urinary sediment of normal individuals. J Clin Invest 2:409–415, 1926
4. Allen RD, David GB, Nomarski G: The Zeiss-Nomarski differential interference equipment for transmitted-light microscopy. Z Wiss Mikrosk 69:193–221, 1969
5. Appel GB, Neu HC: The nephrotoxicity of antimicrobial agents. N Engl J Med 296:663–670, 722–729, 784–787, 1977
6. Arcadi JA: Staining of urinary sediments on a permanent slide: A simple office procedure. J Urol 61:814–818, 1949
7. Behrman RA: Urinary findings before and after a marathon race. N Engl J Med 225:801–802, 1939
8. Beyer-Boon ME, et al: The efficacy of urinary cytology in the detection of urothelial tumors: Sensitivity and specificity of urinary cytology. Urol Res 6:3–12, 1978
9. Bolande RP: Inclusion bearing cells in the urine in certain viral infections. Pediatrics 24:7–12, 1959
10. Brenner BM, Rector FC (eds): The Kidney. Philadelphia: WB Saunders Co, 1976
11. Brody L, Webster MD, Kark RM: Identification of elements of urinary sediment with phase-contrast microscopy. JAMA 206:1,777–1,781, 1979
12. Brody LH, Salladay JR, Armbruster K: Urinalysis and the urinary sediment. Med Clin North Am 55:243–266, 1971
13. Crabbe JGS: "Comet" or "decoy" cells found in urinary sediment smear. Acta Cytol 15:303–305, 1971
14. Dunnil MS: A review of the pathology and pathogenesis of acute renal failure due to acute tubular necrosis. J Clin Pathol 27:2–13, 1974
15. Fletcher AP, et al: The chemical composition and electron microscopic appearance of a protein derived from urinary casts. Biochim Biophys Acta 214:299–308, 1970
16. Free AH, Free HM: Urinalysis in Clinical Laboratory Practice. Cleveland: CRC Press, 1975
17. Friedman IS, Zuckerman S, Cohn TD: The production of urinary casts during the use of cation exchange resins. Am J Med Sci 221:672–677, 1951
18. Haber MH: Interference contrast microscopy for identification of urinary sediments. Am J Clin Pathol 57:316–319, 1972
19. Haber MH: Interference contrast microscopy provides 3-D images of urine sediment. Lab Med 2:9, 10, 47, 1971
20. Haber MH: Urine Casts: Their Microscopy and Clinical Significance, ed 2. Chicago: American Society of Clinical Pathologists, 1976
21. Haber MH: A Primer of Microscopic Urinalysis. Fountain Valley, CA: ICL Scientific, 1978
22. Haber MH, Lindner LE: The surface ultrastructure of urinary casts. Am J Clin Pathol 68:547–552, 1977

23. Haber MH, Lindner LE, Ciofalo LN: Urinary casts after stress. Lab Med 10:351–355, 1979
24. Heptinstall RH: Pathology of the Kidney, ed 2. Boston: Little, Brown & Co, 1974
25. Hudson JB, Dennis AJ, Gerhardt RE: Urinary lipid and the Maltese cross. N Engl J Med 299:586, 1978
26. Imhof PR, et al: Excretions of urinary casts after administration of diuretics. Br Med J 2:199–202, 1972
27. Jones SR, Smith JW, Sanford LP: Localization of urinary tract infections by detection of antibody-coated bacteria in urine sediment. N Engl J Med 20:591–594, 1974
28. Kark RM, et al: A Primer of Urinalysis, ed 2. New York: Harper & Row Pubs, Inc, 1963
29. Kauffman HM Jr, et al: Lymphocytes in urine as an aid in the early detection of renal homograft rejection. Surg Gynecol Obstet 119:25–36, 1969
30. Kern WH: Epithelial cells in urine sediments. Am J Clin Pathol 56:67–72, 1971
31. Kesson AM, Talbott JM, Gyory AZ: Microscopic examination of urine. Lancet 2:809–812, 1978
32. Kierkegaard H, et al: Falsely negative urinary leucocyte counts due to delayed examination. Scand J Clin Lab Invest 40:259–261, 1980
33. Kline TS, Craighead JE: Renal homotransplantation: The cytology of the urine sediment. Am J Clin Pathol 47:802–807, 1967
34. Larcom RC, Carter GH: Erythrocytes in urinary sediment: Identification and normal limits. J Lab Clin Med 33:875–880, 1948
35. Letterne GM: The urinary sediment in renal disease. Med Clin North Am 47:887–901, 1963
36. Lindner LE, Haber MH: Unsuitability of electron microscopic examination of urinary sediment for the diagnosis of amyloidosis: Universal presence of fibrillar proteins in urine containing casts. Am J Clin Pathol 71:40–42, 1979
37. Lindner LE, Jones RN, Haber MH: A specific urinary cast in acute pyelonephritis. Am J Clin Pathol 73:809–811, 1980
38. Lindquist B, Wahlin A: Differential count of urinary leukocytes and renal epithelial cells by phase contrast microscopy. Acta Med Scand 198:505–509, 1975
39. Lippman RW: Urine and the Urinary Sediment, ed 2. Springfield, Ill.: Charles C Thomas, Publisher, 1957
40. Manuel Y, Revillard JP, Betuel H (eds): Proteins in Normal and Pathologic Urine. Baltimore: University Park Press, 1970
41. McKenzie JK, McQueen EG: Immunofluorescent localization of Tamm-Horsfall mucoprotein in human kidney. J Clin Pathol 22:334–339, 1969
42. McQueen EG: Composition of urinary casts. Lancet 1:397–398, 1966
43. McQueen EG, Engel GB: Factors determining the aggregation of urinary mucoprotein. Am J Clin Pathol 19:392–396, 1966
44. Modern Urinalysis: A Guide to the Diagnosis of Urinary Tract Diseases and Metabolic Disorders. Elkhart, IN: Ames Co, 1974
45. Papanicolaou GN: Cytology of urine sediment in neoplasms of the urinary tract. J Urol 57:375–379, 1947
46. Pollak VE, Arbel C: The distribution of Tamm-Horsfall mucoprotein (uromucoid) in the human nephron. Nephron 6:667–672, 1969
47. Riedasch, Ritz E: Antibody coating of urinary tract bacteria. N Engl J Med 299:606, 1978
48. Riggs SA, et al: Plasma cells in urine: Occurrence in multiple myeloma. Arch Intern Med 135:1,245–1,247, 1975
49. Roberts AM: Some effects of exercise on the urinary sediment. J Clin Invest 14:31–33, 1935
50. Rutecki GJ, Goldsmith C, Schreiner GE: Characterization of proteins in urinary casts. N Engl J Med 284:1,049–1,052, 1971
51. Schreiner GE: The identification and clinical significance of casts. Arch Intern Med 99:356–369, 1957
52. Schreiner GE: The urinary sediment. Clin Symp 13:35–48, 1961

53. Schumann GB: Urine Sediment Examination. Baltimore: Williams & Wilkins Co, 1980
54. Schumann GB, Harris S, Henry JB: An improved technic for examining urinary casts and a review of their significance. Am J Clin Pathol 69:18–23, 1978
55. Schumann GB, Palmieri LJ, Jones DB: Differentiation of renal tubular epithelium in renal transplantation cytology. Am J Clin Pathol 67:580–584, 1977
56. Spencer ES, Pedersen I: Hand Atlas of the Urinary Sediment: Bright-Field, Phase-Contrast, and Polarized-Light. Baltimore: University Park Press, 1971
57. Sternheimer R: A supravital cytodiagnostic stain for urinary sediments. JAMA 231:826–832, 1975
58. Sternheimer R, Malbin B: Clinical recognition of pyelonephritis with a new stain for urinary sediments. Am J Med 11:312–323, 1951
59. Sutor AH, Ketelsen UP, Schindera F: Platelets in the urine: Further evidence. Thromb Haemostas 36:647–648, 1976
60. Tamm I, Horsfall FL Jr: A mucoprotein derived from human urine which reacts with influenza, mumps, and Newcastle disease viruses. J Exp Med 95:71–97, 1952
61. Thomas V, Skelokov A, Fraland M: Antibody coated bacteria in the urine and the site of urinary tract infection. N Engl J Med 290:588–590, 1974
62. Tweeddale DN: Urinary Cytology. Boston: Little, Brown & Co, 1977
63. Urine under the Microscope. Nutley, NJ: ROCOM Press, 1973
64. Voogt HJ, Beyer-Boon ME, Brussee JM: The value of phase contrast microscopy for urinary cytology, reliability and pitfalls. Acta Cytol 19:542–546, 1975
65. Winer RL, et al: Ultrastructural examination of urinary sediment: Value in renal amyloidosis. Am. J Clin Pathol 71:36–39, 1979

Index

D

E

F

G

H